NAVIGATING THE NOOSPHERE

THE FORGOTTEN ART OF HEALING

From the Series of *The Teachings of Julian*

NAVIGATING THE NOOSPHERE

THE FORGOTTEN ART OF HEALING

- Book 1 -

Wolfgang Henckert

First ebook edition: May 2021

First paperback edition: July 2021

Second paperback edition: August 2021

Cover Design by Roy-Lee Kitt

ISBN-10 1513685740 (paperback)

ISBN-13 978-1-513-68574-8 (paperback)

ASIN B093YC4K8C (eBook)

www.dadirri-institute.org

ACKNOWLEDGMENTS

The manuscripts to this series spent many months, if not years, in the making. The process was oscillating nicely between trying to find the words for what I would like to term "downloads", and understanding that there are equally enough books in this world to support some, if not all, of the ideas and notions I have collected over time. Yet, I found myself lovingly supported by family and friends on various physical, energetic, spiritual and consciousness levels. The journey of this is humbling and empowering, it deconstructs you and it reconstructs you, placing you on a different footing each time you enter the proverbial rabbit hole.

Despite this, there is a consistency to the process that is of otherworldly nature. In a way, I am following my Higher Self, and as I do, I am brought into contact with those that equally do, or equally did prior to me, patiently waiting for me to literally raise my vibrations even further. This process does not need to be pretty, but it needs to be truthful. This is quite unpleasant when old parameters, conditions, situations, people, connections, or even opportunities slowly but surely fall away. Mostly, this was not out of my own volition, but a consequence of *resonance*. This is a peculiar concept for many that is difficult to understand - until it literally happens under your nose.

I am thus particularly in resonant harmony with my wife, my children, and my family for allowing me the time and space to mature into finding and raising my own light, much of which is a mere reflection of theirs. Similarly, many friends have spent considerable time in reading this manuscript with many critiques and interjections. I thank you all for your feedback, your corrections, your misunderstandings of and your perspectives on how to improve this text.

∞

May this work find its way to you, the reader, and inspire you to entrain your life to more light and harmony.

∞

PREFACE

This book has been in the making for as long as I have been in the making. Many different interests, ideas, and experiences flow together to weave a tapestry of awareness which gave rise to plenty of increasingly complex and mind-bending insights that find their expression in *The Teachings of Julian*.

When I started to pen down the contents of this book, I saw myself – amongst many other - as a so-called healer, despite my complex relationship with the term. On a certain level of explanation, I believed I could make a difference in the lives of people by helping them reframe their illnesses and perhaps walk a different path.

However, my experiences in energy world have brought me to a point where I was confronted with my, albeit, *unrealised* true energy. In order to bring these insights into this world, you need to raise your hand on the 'other' side. You embark on a path of moving closer towards the realisation of your true and Higher Self. It also gave me a new understanding about my past decades of relentless study and gathering of knowledge across a wide and diverse spectrum of knowledge areas. I also came to understand that the message in this book can and will take care of itself. In order to get out of the way of the Divine Light and out of the way of the message, I was assigned the pseudonym of *Julian*, so that people may see the message and not the messenger.

This book is a journey of sorts, and for those of you who instinctively grasp the truth of my writings, please be encouraged to continue on your journey to feel, think, and live.

For those of you who are a beginning reader perhaps, please be encouraged to start where you are, with what you have, and understand that your life *is* spiritual in nature, even though it may feel everything but Spiritual.

To all of us, may we all be encouraged to allow the Light even more. May we find the strength to reconnect, the ability to let go of past trauma, and allow the Light as supreme reality of all dimensions. May we all rise in strength that is rooted in a humble understanding of our own intransigence when engaging in that which we call our reality.

Understand that everything is changeable, and it starts with yourself. Reality beckons to be created.

∞

CONTENTS

INTRODUCTION

This book is about things that matter. It is about what you see as material. Yet, it is not about matter at all.

It is about energy. It is about what energises you and drives you to live your life, among other matter that matters to you. However, somehow, it is not about energy either.

It is about consciousness. It is about those vibrations and frequencies that condense into any other form, shape or condition of energy which we would usually call anything *but* consciousness.

In its own way, this book is about your career as a human being on this earth, the way you deal with what you describe to others and yourself as *reality*: the way you are embroiled in that reality, and how this reality can hurt you, impact on you, stifle you, throw you; the extent to which you believe you are in charge of your own affairs, your body and mind, how much control you exert over others and the objects in your perceived external environment; and about how you will move forward from here. What kind of labyrinth are you pursuing in your life, which layers upon layers of what you call reality are you bringing forth; what kind of ghost-in-a-machine are you, and how much do you identify with that which we so easily call the 'I', the 'me', my 'Self'? What did, or do you currently make of your embodiment on earth?

The 'I', the 'me', the 'Self': these are all wonderful constructs that allow us to blame ourselves for not achieving what countless self-help books sell you and tell you. We think that perhaps there is something wrong with ourselves, more than we thought, that our wrongness is beyond the scope of this or that book. So we buy the next book, and as long as we keep searching, we actually believe that we need to improve ourselves even more. So we try more, we attempt to reach deeper, to look further; we challenge ourselves to think more out of the box. However, trying to improve ourselves is a typical Western way of thinking. It might have to do with Western civilisation's concept of process optimisation. Because the Western worldview is one of being incomplete, permanently under construction like a building, we learn to be in a constant state of imperfection, something we continuously need to atone for. It is an inflation-proof way of selling self-help books. Forever.

Understand that this is not correct. This notion fills churches and sells books, but you are selling yourself short. This is also not what the Divine intends for you. It is time this came to an end, starting today! It is time that we honour and cherish the light within each one of us, and that we begin living a life that celebrates this light and the unique embodiment that each one of us is.

> *Slow down, and witness yourself as you navigate what you call your life.*

As you nosedive into your future, this book will inspire you to *feel* deeper, *think* further, and *live* more consciously and conscientiously. I challenge you to combine this book with the lessons of your own life. I challenge you to acknowledge it all, put it all on the table - just to equally let it all go in in one big swoop and to bring new and fresh lessons into your personal future. Lessons that will catapult your growth and success, and that will make you a part of this book.

Consider opening up to all the possibilities beyond your current outlook or outreach in life. Allow things to happen, to fall into place, to transform your environment and to transform you. Who would you be if you were to allow this? Perhaps you are afraid you couldn't say no to all the choices you would suddenly be presented with, or perhaps the process of 'going shopping' will take you too far from your original departure point?

> *May you all rise to the occasion!*

Look up from your busy daily lives, take a few minutes to look back, possibly even read this book in smaller chunks. May you find this book helpful on your path of healing yourself and honouring the Divine within yourself! Regularly return to your own book of life, and consider how you could inspire others to love, think, feel, or stretch further. Your book will be based on you, on your success and how modulating your consciousness, moving through an endless and limitless sea of energy – where everything is possible – and tapping this world the right way will allow you to move forward differently in your current life.

And for this, I wish you the most heartfelt of inspiration to grow and thrive on your insights, and bringing the Light into your life.

Much blessings, love and success.

∞

NOOMON I

∞

IMAGINE

I magine.

We will start our journey with a short meditation.

Imagine a vast ocean. All you can see is water, stretching to the horizon in every direction. The water is deep and blue and calm. There is a beautiful and protective sky above, with a few clouds here and there; it is a beautiful day in a watery paradise. Focus on taking deep and fulfilling breaths, nothing else. If your mind wanders off, come back to your breathing. Listen to your breathing as you take in this picture of water all around you. Perhaps you can even smell the sea. Do this for as long as you like!

Immerse yourself in this picture for a few minutes; try to think of nothing else except this picture, and your breathing. You are surrounded by the panorama of the ocean. Follow your breath from the tip of your nose, through your nose, into your throat, into your lungs, and then all the way back out through your mouth or your nose. When you exhale, feel how the air from your nose moves over your upper lip; feel the warmth of the air on your face. Do this for a few minutes.

Keep breathing calmly, stay in the here and now, and imagine you are an island rising from the depths below, being born into this endless expanse of water. You are here. You are *you*. Think of the waters around you as the collective energies of other people: your ancestors, friends and relatives, and strangers near and far. Slowly, you will see other islands in these waters, some nearer, others off in the distance. All these islands create movement, tides in the water; some consciously, others just by being there. This great ocean of energies from previous generations and the people now on earth can be overwhelming. Not only that, but soon you realise that the air you are breathing is actually at the bottom of a sea of oxygen and nitrogen that rests in layers above the waters you were born into. Surely, we are dwellers in the deep: there are just so many layers to this world...

So here you are, slowly making your ascent, steadily growing from a tiny spit of land, the waves washing over you repeatedly, to a majestic island, with impressive coastlines, elaborate jungles, waterfalls, cliffs, desert, meadows, pastures, beaches, rocky outcrops; the possibilities are endless. However, you also realise that these waves keep crashing against your shorelines. Over here, they create beautiful beaches; on another part of your shoreline, they may create steep and slippery reefs and whatever *you*, the island, feature.

However, you cannot avoid these waters that surround you; they keep forming and transforming your coastline. Surely, they erode your substance, and they may deposit other people's debris (their emotions, beliefs, views, and opinions) on your coastlines. Positive thinking will not spare you from the onslaught of these incessant and unruly waves. The constant intrusion of the waves may create bad weather on your island, despite the lush vegetation, the unicorns in the meadows, or the quantum jumps of the elves in the magical forest; despite the abysses of hopelessness, the dark pits of loneliness.

This is your *noosphere*, your world, your individual environment, where only you can thrive, or suffer. This is the sphere of your consciousness, where you collect and harvest information, like a farmer domesticating and farming his land. Ideally, this process will increase the flow of information and energy; it will mimic the universal ebb and flow of 'frequency', 'vibration', 'energy'; unlocking the flow of resources into and about your life as an island.

The constellation of all resources, whether available or potential, the way you feel about everything (including yourself), and the outside factors you find yourself confronted with: all of this is a part of what you are. You are at the centre of *your* spider web, always, whether you feel upbeat and in control or like a victim in your own life. It is a unique constellation that resembles no other, no matter how similar they may seem. In addition, this constellation, this web, will feel so overwhelmingly true to you that you have little room for doubt about the validity of everything or anything. And yet, you should examine everything. Understand that an imagined lion feels as real to your stress centres as would a real lion. That which you are so afraid of or worried about loses its power once you entertain the possibility that it is really just an imaginary threat. Once you start looking at everything in your life with a more refined understanding about its true *spiritual* nature, you start to worry less about that which you cannot change, and you start to appreciate that which you experience: this world is an experiential world. Experience everything, not blindly, not wildly, but through awareness, taking ownership and integrating your faculties. Experience the world, not like an actor on a stage, but by seeing the so-called objective reality out there as an expression of Spirit, tailored to the way you see yourself.

Ultimately, one of the biggest illusion we need to overcome is our feeling of being an island in an ocean, of being separate from the energetic ocean of consciousness around us, of rising above the waters. And when we overcome this illusion, we experience a universe of Creation that is endlessly beautiful. Our blessings are abundantly dispersed across our noosphere; we often just need to take a moment to calm down and look around us. Engage with the world, explore your island, appreciate Creation, worship the ground you walk on, think of yourself as co-Creator, create your island, shape it and bless it, investigate all your fears, overcome those you can overcome, clear the rubble off your track, the weeds off your land, the destructive energies from your coastlines, and travel safely while observing with more compassion and less attachment.

Create wisely, and witness Creation.

Feel. Think. Live.

∞

11

NOOMON II
∞
THE WEB OF LIFE

Here you are – a newly created island, and there is *so* much to discover! Will you ever have enough time? What if this happened, or that? What if I did this, or that? The list of possibilities that might influence you on your growth path is endless. One thing is for sure, though – your island will eventually disappear.

This concept of a gradual diminishing of substance or order is referred to as *entropy* in physics, and it has its roots in the Second Law of Thermodynamics. It derives from the simple principle that heat from an object or environment tends to dissipate toward objects or environments that are less hot, until the objects or environments involved reach a state of equal temperature.

Your island will be subjected to an incessant onslaught of waters from all sides and above. Yes, they will nourish certain areas, for example your rivers, your lakes, your forests and all your vegetation, but these waters will also erode your coastline; rock faces will turn into sand over many years and mountainous areas into nothing but hilly outcrops. And just like the wheels of your car will lose their rubber coating due to abrasion on the road's surface, the concentrated energy of your rocky material, for all its solid appearance and splendour will be lost to the environment.

Entropy refers to a state of disorder and probability, where disorder simply is more probable than order: when you toss around a number of kids' building blocks in the air, they are highly unlikely to arrange themselves into a discernible shape or structure, such as a heart, a house, or even a geometric figure such as a circle, a triangle, a cube or a pyramid. Similarly, why would all atoms and molecules in the universe not spread out evenly, but cluster in huge swaths of ordered arrangements we call 'matter', an 'organ', or an 'organism'? Entropy refers to the observation that devolve from orderly states to disorderly states, and that such disorder is more probable than the ordered arrangement.

The human body, for example, is such a non-entropic, or *negentropic* system: if you compare the cells of our body to the analogy of Lego pieces, what are the chances that, if you throw 37-odd trillion cells into the air, a human body will emerge? Although your island is shaped by outside forces, *something* in you creates a kind of order for which we currently have no explanation, and which we call life.

The discovery of the principle of entropy had far-reaching ramifications for a large number of sciences, and the subject has been discussed and investigated by a great many thinkers and researchers. Entropy turns out to be a highly versatile and malleable concept, and over the years, thinking on entropy has gone in many different directions. In general, the process of lowering entropy has the effect of increasing the energy, power, or information available to an entity. In the human body there is more discernible structure and less entropy than there would be if one were to liquefy the body in a big container. Equally, there is less entropy in a bowl of vegetables than if we were to put it all in a blender and mix it; the information content in a body, or an intact vegetable for that matter, is higher than in its constituent parts.

> *What could this mean for energy medicine principles and practices?*

When the concept of entropy is used in the realm of consciousness studies, the lowering of entropy is equated with *more consciousness*, and would allow for spiritual growth while increasing the quality of consciousness. Entropy has been successfully and repeatedly used to explain biological and spiritual evolution.

> *Consciousness seems to be the commonality upon which all maturation is based, and the totality of all development can be explained as different expressions of the same thing.*

Therefore, your island has certain negentropic characteristics; as an ordered system, it has more information content, and thus consciousness, than a disordered or random system. What are these negentropic characteristics?

∞

Information theory is an important development in cosmology and system studies. What is the nature and dynamics of the *information density* and *information content* of the universe on the one hand, and our activities within the universe on the other? What are the parameters that successfully differentiate between matter and consciousness? What is this state we call life? Is the earth alive? Is *everything* alive? How do we define and distinguish a living organism from its seemingly material environment? Research in complexity, chaos, information, and systems theory all point to an uncanny order within chaos.

But what about meaning within chaos?

The movement of water drops in a cloud is chaotic when looked at from close proximity, but more orchestrated when seen from further away. What about the play of colours at sunset? Is this perceived 'order' contained in the data, or does it take something like consciousness to make sense of it? This area of research is complex and has much to learn from quantum physics and its paradoxes.

What is reality?

When we add it all together, it seems that the larger system, into which we all are embedded, is conscious, aware, and possibly evolving. We might just be an individuated unit of consciousness, a fragment of the larger system. This viewpoint, incidentally, serves as a basic teaching in many religious and philosophical traditions around the world, and it is still vital in the 21st century:

All reality frames and everything contained in them are a part of the same system of consciousness – we are all connected.

17

We have thus found another characteristic of your island: it is embedded in a *sea of consciousness*, aware of its own existence, constantly interacting with its environment on various levels. Important here is the insight that a living organism receives and gives repeated feedback from and to its environment. These reiterative feedback loops allow systems to self-optimise, to increase or decrease activity, to continually lower entropy by self-regulation, self-optimisation, to express themselves using all available resources to increase the informational content of systems and sub-systems, as well as the interactions shaped by those systems with their environments.

So then, how do we actually do that?

Unlike a rock in the desert that slowly succumbs to entropy and eventually disintegrates, a *dissipative system* persistently maintains its shape, form, or identity, because it is neither a closed system nor an open system, but one which maintains a flow of energy through itself. The human body is such a dissipative system, as it is able to maintain energy flows, from sources such as food, water, and air, and even control environmental stimuli and cognitive processes. A lot of research has shown that the dynamics of the intra-systemic interactions of such dissipative systems lean toward tipping points, rather than equilibrium. The easiest way to explain this is with an analogy: If I was blind, and you were tasked with describing a painting in a museum to me, how would you do that? If you were to use five thousand, five million, or fifty million words to describe the picture, would you be able to explain to me precisely what you were seeing? Perhaps you could take the picture apart and tell me about each and every colour pixel, starting in the top left corner and ending in the bottom right corner. Would that work? Modern Gestalt psychology says, no, this is not possible – the Gestalt is more than its constituent parts. Similarly, if we took an organism apart, atom by atom, molecule by molecule, and reassembled it, would it become a living organism again? Probably not.

This is a problem for science!

If you account for all constituent parts of an entity, and after meticulous reassembly the entity is still not functioning as before, then there is clearly something missing. However, the instruments and measurements of science are unable to account for this missing part(s). It seems that complex systems break the beautiful, mechanistic simplicity of reductionism. How can simple conditions generate complex outcomes that cannot be predicted by the sum of the constituent parts? This conundrum forced scientists to contemplate the thing that many of us fear most – chaos.

The orchestrated movement of a flock of birds in flight is a classic example of how a swarm can *act intelligently without a central intelligence.* Research into swarm intelligence has shown, however, that a centralised intelligence is not necessary to coordinate the entire flock. All that is needed is that each bird maintains a constant distance from its neighbours while flying in the same general direction Simple rules can thus generate emergent, complex behaviour. Similar self-organising patterns are observed almost everywhere, from ants engaged in organised labour, to fish swimming in fantastic and complex shoals, to interstellar spiral galaxy formations.

So how do complex systems generate simple outcomes? Let's take a living organism such as your body; its trillions of cells all work together to keep you alive, yet your body acts as a single unit. Something happens when large numbers of cells come together and interact with each other. This interaction gives rise to an emergent phenomenon called self-organisation. This also means that an investigation of a single cell does not reveal its ability to work together with other cells and systems that eventually form your body. Starting out with a single cell, we are unable to predict what a complex system, like each one of us is, will evolve into. Mixing together ten million liver cells will not make a liver, despite our best intentions. The concept of *emergence,* how components of a system eerily develop collective properties or patterns out of their interactions with each other and in relation to each other, are not reducible to the system's constituent components.

One of the ramifications of this is that the biological mechanism of DNA cannot explain an *apparent* transfer of information across biological boundaries.

What??

19

Living systems engage in self-sustaining processes, engage in intricate networks of production processes that interact and inter-depend, where the output of countless processes serve as the input to countless other processes. So intertwined is the complex of processes, producing or transforming energy from food, air, water, information, and so on, that the network at least *seems* self-sustaining; the network can maintain itself. Within a living system, the most obvious characteristic is *self-organisation*, the creation of a boundary between what the system is to itself, and what it is or represents in the bigger context of its environment. For a single cell, this would be the cell membrane, but for a complex organism like yourself, would that be your skin? Your belief system about yourself and others? The language you speak? The religion you follow?

Living systems consist of numerous parts that exist and function together to ensure the survival and reproduction of the entire system. From this dialogue that living systems have with their environment, emergent phenomena stemming from such practices of interaction lead to a new order which is discernible, yet, when seen from a higher perspective, is nothing but another component in another, bigger system, participating in the emergence of yet another, higher order.

The field of epigenetics has shown that the human embeddedness into, and interaction with, its environment cannot possibly be explained by a reductionist biological model of structure-function relationships. Living organisms are not just physical entities in a physical environment; the perception of the outside world and inside life of the organism adds to the expression or suppression of certain genetic features. The self-reference and self-perception of the organism are critical determinants of evolution, something that Darwin's theory completely ignored. In addition, the attempts to integrate perception, and those activities that stem from perception, into the adaptation to, and interaction with, the organism's environment, have led to new approaches that move decisively beyond mechanical determinism and dependency on genetic information to account for the negentropic factors that characterise living systems.

That said, there is currently no scientific consensus on how to delineate the observed energies, magnetic fields, optical messaging, or remote interactions, for example between humans, or humans and animals, or even humans and matter. To the physicist, this poses enormous problems, in that the universe is not what the sum of our theories predicts (despite the elegance of those theories); there seem to be as yet unquantified, untestable, postulated fields that connect us all. A mere hundred years ago we spoke of the *ether*, and many other thinkers followed suit and postulated a form of *biofield*. The current biomechanical model used in mainstream medical interventions is one example where this field is assumed not to exist, while any effect that could point in the direction of such a field is currently dismissed under the sweeping umbrella term of *placebo effect*.

The self-generating patterns in networks are defining characteristics of all living systems. This insight is essential in understanding the extent to which such systems operate beyond thermodynamic equilibrium. The dynamics of such systems is non-linear, and specifically includes the spontaneous emergence of new, different, higher forms of order. The inflow and outflow of energy in such systems should be treated as a given in dissipative structures, as it enables us to explain positive feedback cycles which stimulate the system beyond its capacity to withstand stress and bifurcate, branching off into a new state of order with new structures and possibly even new components.

Bifurcations happen at critical points of instability, and are one of the most important concepts of the new understanding of life. Countless trillions of grains of sand heap up to form a sand dune, and they will pile up until the dune collapses. The system collapses at a critical point of instability; the sides of the dune start to slide, sand runs down and forms a new base upon which new grains are piled up: the system establishes a new order and structure. This spontaneous emergence of order is called *self-organisation*, and has been recognised as the dynamic origin of development, learning, creativity and evolution. Living systems develop and evolve continuously; life constantly reaches out in novel ways. Positive feedback loops reiterate and exponentially exacerbate initial stresses in the system, eventually rendering it unable to absorb shocks and re-establish the original equilibrium. A critical point of instability is inevitable, bifurcation occurs, and the system develops, grows, and adapts.

∞

Your island will of course be shaped by other forms of positive feedback loops too: such as waves crashing onto your shorelines and eroding your soil. All in all, your island will develop vegetation and beautiful landscapes from positive feedback loops that collapse from time to time, only to find a more stable or optimal base from which to develop yet again.

When you remove the term *stasis* from your internal dictionary and replace it with *dynamics* you allow a more holistic view to enter your life. Homeostasis is traded as the gold standard of biological equilibrium, yet the term stasis really is a misnomer. Everything is in a state of *negotiated balance*, and all living systems, from the smallest to the biggest, continually engage in this balancing act. To merely maintain that this is a state of static balance is not only wrong; it creates a wrong view of oneself, the world, and the dynamic integrity of everything.

When you remove the term *hierarchy* and replace it with *cycle*, you break old patterns of thinking, feeling, and acting. Hierarchy presupposes inequality. This is particularly unfortunate in that it creates division where there are none, and it creates suffering where there is none. Unlike the traditional understanding of the Tower of Babel recount as about a mutual misunderstanding that thwarted collective ambition, it seems fit to introduce that the notion of hierarchy leads to notions of supremacy. It has given rise to countless ravaging wars over the past centuries. Our overuse of such terms has created a world that makes people sick, a world that impoverishes nations, and that allows us to think of ourselves as the epitome of Creation.

Growth happens when your system can no longer tolerate stress. However, you don't just break down, though you may do at first. Instead, you find a new, elevated level of stability. You then proceed to grow, learn, emerge stronger through reiterative processes that positively influence and reinforce the newly found balance.

You are tasked to find out how *you* adapt to change. What do *you* need to enable change? More security? More safety? More money?

Which factors in your life force you to stay put, and which factors force you out of your comfort zone?

Try to identify the push and pull factors in your life and how you react to them. Look for small and large patterns of interaction.

Start with yourself, your family, your neighbourhood, your peer group, and move on to your city, your country, the world.

∞

NOOMON III
∞
THE SCAFFOLDING OF LIFE

Cognition, the process of knowing, seems to be central to a living organism; it is crucial to the processes of self-generation and self-perpetuation. Living systems are dissipative structures; we handle energies in a different way than, say, a rock in the desert. We need to recognise that cognition is a *process* and a *strategy* by which the system maintains its dissipative nature: cognition is the very process of life.

Life and cognition are inseparably connected.

This understanding of cognition is a radical expansion of the traditional concept of body and mind; it means that cognition involves the entire process of life, not just the mind. Western philosophy has been greatly influenced by the idea of the division between body and mind, as epitomised by the works of Descartes, and his theories enabled the flourishing of reductionism as the basis for modern science. So the consequences of introducing cognition into the biological processes of living are profound, in that we not only experience, but we also think and reflect, we make value judgements, we hold beliefs, we communicate, and we act with intentions, all this is part of the overarching process of *self-awareness*.

The scientific discourse of the past two hundred years has highlighted the fact that knowledge about the world can be gained in several ways. On the one hand there is the scientific approach, grounded in evaluating, measuring, and experimenting in an effort to increase objectivity and accuracy. On the other hand, we have subjective and internal knowledge, which includes feelings, and intuition. These considerations are important in maintaining a perspective on human experiences where *health* and *illness* have both objective and subjective meaning for the individual. These issues surface in how patients *feel* about themselves, their illness, and their resulting coping strategies, and how these all relate to more or less dysfunctional metacognitive beliefs about themselves or the world.

We don't just blindly react to outside conditions and forces. As living organisms, we are not passive expressions of gene activity; we construct ourselves from the confines of our DNA and our environments during our development. Of course, we can suffer a dislocated shoulder through physical trauma to the shoulder area, but equally we can store emotions and psychological trauma in visceral or fascial tissue. Whatever happens to, with, or because of our belief system has an element of cognition and consciousness.

The extent to which non-physical affects can masquerade as physical symptoms – to which modern healthcare would normally respond with manual or chemical interventions – has been demonstrated by many studies in recent years and has given rise to the research field of epigenetics. A good example is how depression may affect the length of telomeres in white blood cells and mitochondrial functioning. Telomere length is a chromosomal indicator for how often cells can replicate. With every replication – for example, as old cells die off and are replaced by new cells – the telomere on the chromosome shortens. Once the telomeres are unable to shorten any further, the cell can no longer replicate.

Such studies have shown that, for example, men who were inclined to internalise their emotions also show an increased shortening of their telomere length. Given at the additional effects of lifestyle, depression, stress, and secondary disease states such as cholesterol, cardiovascular diseases and high blood pressure, these patients might present with anything from lower back pains, visceral abdominal pains, chronic headaches, frozen shoulder, or a plethora of other symptoms. The questions we need to ask are:

> *Why is this happening? How many other, if not all, biological processes are influenced by cognition, which we are often not even aware of? What does this mean for consciousness and health?*

Functional medicine has shown that gut health, inflammation, and brain function are closely related. This is remarkably similar to the approach of complementary and alternative medicine modalities, where the brain-body connection is presented differently to the way mainstream medicine currently sees it. A study on gut health suggested that the gut biome can influence the cognition and behaviour of individuals, while the nervous system can directly influence the microbiome. This contradicts everything that biology and medicine has taught for the past 1,000 years. Surprisingly, mindfulness can reduce physical inflammation and reduce the frequency and severity of chronic migraine. It seems that non-mechanical and non-molecular concepts such as epigenetics, metacognition, stress, and feelings can act as critical success factors within the traditional setting of medicine.

What happened? Did the market change? What is the effect of this on the principles and practice of medicine?

∞

Cognition is defined as the activity of the living network that focuses on two distinct features, namely that of *self-renewal* and that of *creating new structures*. Living systems continually generate themselves by co-evolving their interdependent components whilst maintaining their pattern of organisation. Where, and whenever, such a system is forming structural connections to, and relationships with, its environment, the plethora of recurrent interactions trigger structural changes within or around the system. Cognition is an activity that positively reinforces connecting to the environment, eventually leading the system towards bifurcation, innovation, adaptation, and evolution. It is precisely such structural coupling that allows one to deduce the distinction between living and non-living systems.

Such intimate couplings with the environment are an indicator of *learning systems*. The system interacts with its environment cognitively, actively incorporating structural changes in the environment into its internal structures or adjusting the way it interacts with the environment in future. Given enough time and opportunity, such systems will co-evolve and adapt to each other in a very specific and individual way. At any given point in time, the structure and its behaviour represents a record of the system's coupling with the environment, and how the system is determined by its structure. The organism is generating itself and its own structures as a response to feedback received on all and any levels, the totality of which is cognition. The ensuing dialogue between individual structure and environmental influences, and the interdependence between the system and outside forces, develop along stochastic trajectories:

The behaviour of living systems is determined by the extent to which it is free; what determines living systems causally, is simultaneously an expression of autonomy.

As opposed to being simply *reactive*, a living system employs cognition to filter environmental triggers, to allow for selective feedback, and possibly pre-empt system collapse by anticipating what factor represents a perturbation or danger, and to which extent such a trigger allows for structural changes of the system or organism. However, positive feedback often undermines the system's ability to compensate, leading to an earlier collapse. Imagine a coral reef. When conditions are very favourable, the coral will grow faster, multiply quicker, grow more branches on the reef; positive feedback from the environment such as more food, ideal water temperatures, and low levels of disturbance, allow the system to grow and bifurcate quicker than under adverse conditions. A living system employs cognition to filter environmental triggers; not all triggers are worth reacting to. This allows for *selective feedback*, and potentially pre-empts bifurcation by anticipating what factor represents a perturbation, and to what extent a trigger allows for structural changes of the system or organism. Living systems thus create their own realities. This is why you could be triggered by something or somebody, and you create elaborate mechanisms, explanations, emotions, behaviours, defences, beliefs, and other structural couplings with your environment, such as illness, a pain, a 'blind eye' or a 'deaf ear', to avoid the factor which you were afraid of to begin with.

In any case, your process of cognition is an emergent property or pattern of interaction between highly complex systems, which means that the systems don't create cognition, but the interplay between them does. However, it seems that cognition does not equal consciousness: the former is an epiphenomenon, the latter is not. Cognition is thus a self-generating network pattern, and is the result of interaction with others and the environment that enable positive feedback loops to stimulate the system towards bifurcation.

Attempting to establish a relationship between the principles of entropy discussed earlier and how such principles act on closed systems – and the related study of open, dissipative systems, their cognitive properties, the process of bifurcation, and the reinterpretation of all such activities in terms of information - shows us that information transfer between biological systems can be used as an explanation for the observed physical universe, including the realities of quantum mechanics.

> *Your island is self-aware, self-generating, and cognitively interacts with the environment. You maintain borders, you maintain identity, and you maintain internal organisation, despite the waters eating away at your periphery.*

For many people, the process of a *meaningful* life is defined in terms of information; life is a process of lowering entropy, a process of raising the information content or the information quality within one's own life or the higher order system. The lowering of entropy and the raising of information content or quality is a reciprocal process; one will not work without the other. The logical inference from such reasoning is that consciousness is affected by the quality of that information.

> *What, then, are the consequences?*

∞

From a biological perspective, human life has conquered most of the environmental niches on this planet; we have not specialised into a particular ecological niche, precisely because we are so adaptive and resilient. It is, however, exactly this non-specialisation which prevents us from recognising the damage we are creating to ecological niches which, incidentally, are all inhabited by specialised species and systems. Thus a holistic self-understanding has ecological consequences in that it embeds cognition into the very process of living an – ideally – healthy life.

Entropy will prevail when systems isolate and close themselves off. Such systems cannot exchange matter, information, and energy with their environments any longer and must, necessarily, degenerate. Human beings would do so quite rapidly if they didn't constantly take in new matter, energy, or information from the environment. All living organisms thus generate order (and thus reduce entropy) within themselves. This is not an endless process, and at some stage they do succumb to entropy. For the living organism this means biological death.

Human beings need to maintain their dissipative condition by allowing a continuous exchange between themselves and their environment.

On a bigger scale, but by a similar flow of principles, one can observe that fundamentalisms block new ideas, closed societies block new development and innovation, and closed biotic communities prevent new gene flows to be introduced with the consequence that such systems descend into entropic states more rapidly than comparative open systems. Similarly, individuals that feel unsafe will resort to fight-flight-freeze-fawn responses in all forms and shapes, threatened societies may pull up walls or increase policing activities, and Nations close the borders and talk about National policies, law and order, or, as a last resort, of the "good old times".

The application of *cognitive authority* to a living system has a profound effect on our daily lives; there is a reason why each individual life looks and feels the way it does. Yes, we can suffer material physical consequences due to a car accident, and these can be treated with a variety of modern medical interventions. However, when it comes to somatised emotions – dealing with trauma, life circumstances, adverse conditions, chronic pain, serious illness, and so on – one should ask the question *why* such elements are present in one's life. For some or other reason, the individual has established certain structural relationships with his or her environment simply because the environment serves a purpose. These relationships can take many shapes and forms, and naturally there are plenty of psychological mechanisms at play, but seen from a standpoint of cognition, the organism is either failing and dying, or succeeding and living, irrespective of how warped the life path and coupling to the environment is.

Personal health demands that we respond in a committed way to, and live consistently with, the drive to remain within the ambit of a dissipative structure. It demands that we act as self-generating systems, open and ready to embrace this life. This requires a tremendous degree of self-responsibility – which acts as a positive feedback loop – as well as self-integrity, which is the congruence between inner and outer values. The result of this is an *inner freedom* that allows for holistic health and living the creative vision of ourselves.

Life seems rooted in complexity theory, showing us on a daily basis how there can be order and disorder alike within such complex systems. The way and extent to which a living system organises itself as a configuration, a pattern of relationships between its constituent components, equates to a pattern of self-organisation. These are the system's essential characteristics. However, one needs to keep in mind that such patterned interactions are created continually, in response to a plethora of influences, and create a cycle of cognition and self-creation. The dynamic interactivity of a system, its process of living, and the countless structural couplings and embeddedness within the environment, are thus cognitive processes, and effectively enable us to painlessly abandon the tradition of body-mind dualism. Why? Because cognition is embedded in all life processes, not just the mind, not just the brain, not just a specific organ or cell!

When cognition is defined in terms of self-generating networks, it implies a novel approach to interpreting interactivity between a system and its environment. It is when cognition turns into reflective consciousness, and involves an ability to abstract, to hold mental images which in turn allow individuals, groups, and societies, to formulate and express goals, strategies and beliefs, that we can interpret such functions as evolutionary strategies which have enabled the development of language and communication, and with it, the development of groups, communities and societies, and nations. When humans share language and communication, they also interpret life similarly. Common understanding leads to a common identity, which may sometimes bind those individuals together. Language and communication are a special form of coupling between living organisms that exceed the mere transmission of information. The fact that such coupling is mutual is an indication that recurrent interaction between living organisms allows both organisms to change and adapt, to co-evolve and re-self-generate. Communication is thus a mutual trigger for structural change!

How do you communicate with yourself, with your spouse and children, with friends or family members, and with other people across the globe?

All structural change gives rise to more or less conscious experiences, which in turn give rise to thought, conceptual thought, reflective consciousness, families, groups, communities, and societies. However, as much as such cognitive phenomena are non-material, they are embodied by physical structures. They are emergent phenomena of complex, bifurcating systems. The process of living is inseparably intertwined with the structures and patterns which give rise to such processes!

The human desire to shape the world and realise ideas and concepts has resulted in marvellous and ingenious pieces of engineering and constructions that are unique to the human condition. Whether these ideas have succeeded or failed, our actions in realising ideas reflect who we are. The intricate relationship between human endeavours to make sense of the world by imposing theories of science, and methods of research, and the development of technology is punctuated with repeated failure. At one time or another science has postulated that we will never be able to fly, or that trains travelling faster than 20km/h would be detrimental to the health of the passengers. It would be prudent to believe that modern science is fallible, despite the best of intentions, methods, reasoning, or conclusions. One of the most important reasons for this is that our paradigms – worldviews – often define us and that which we deem possible.

∞

Worldviews are formed by the accumulated experiences of people who participate in the same cultural or sub-cultural environments, and constitute a collective, abstract body of personal experiences. However, worldviews also constitute the paradigms – the way of doing things - within which people solve problems, approach unknown issues, or develop methods by which such concepts are evaluated. Worldviews contain strategies and defence mechanisms. They contain assumptions, assertions and abstractions of all kinds of practical and conceptual issues. This does not mean that worldviews are always positive, or inevitably lead to higher development for those who adhere to them.

Worldviews tend to change, over time, due to the ongoing dynamics of their evolving strategies to solve problems, and the persistence of such problems, the convergence of new discoveries – such as quantum physics – the raising of morale from finding a solution to euthanasia, or philosophical dilemmas such as the rights of the unborn. Given enough momentum, worldviews change starting from the fringes of society, where current values and methodologies are questioned and put to the test, where artists stretch the tastes and sensibilities of their audience. The mainstream core of society tends to adopt new values much later. Very much like the universe expanding at its fringes and being stable at the core, so societies maintain a balance between the avant-garde and mainstream. Often the avant-garde is ridiculed amidst a celebration or resurgence of mainstream ideas and notions.

Worldviews allow people to live their lives *without reflection*; they allow people the spontaneity to do things rather than to think and reflect about them. As practical as such a system of norms and values may be, it repeatedly leads to circumstance where existing norms and values have a certain empirical value, while preventing new, incoming and relevant values to get their fair chance of being tested and explored. Meanwhile *metaphysical thought* is an approach to solving problems that current worldviews cannot succeed in solving because there is just no single, adequate and sufficient way of *knowing*. It tells us that many issues find new and different values when explained by metaphysical science simply because all our current worldviews are inadequate in explaining the nature and extent of the universe, this world, our identity, our person, human nature, and the relationship we have with our environments. Metaphysics reaches from the most intellectually abstracted form right down to the quantum level of action and interaction between us and our immediate or distant environment.

The way we describe our world is an expression of the way we see our world, what we believe in, and what we value in our culture, heritage, sciences, religion, art, identity.

Allowing change is a highly personal and psychological process. Change which is perceived as threatening to our identity is more likely to be opposed and rejected than change which we perceive as enriching, nurturing, liberating and empowering. Enriching our views on the physical, emotional and metaphysical nature of ourselves and everything around is like asking for a new, and if not all-encompassing, at least a more encompassing understanding of what is, what can be, and what would be.

This could lead us to see *illness* as the inability to maintain a dissipative structure. In addition, the increasing numbers of esoteric approaches to healthcare over the last fifty years have one significant common denominator: *energy.* The human organism is a self-referential system where *health* is an emergent property of complexity. As dissipative systems, we are supposed to manage our energy flow to ensure internal organisation. The extent to which modern medical science is grappling with this issue is evidenced by how concepts such as *bioenergetics, placebo, metacognition,* and *epigenetics* have been introduced to, and applied in, medical research. While placebo refers to a positive clinical outcome that cannot be attributed to the physical properties of a specific treatment, it is still poorly understood, and randomised controlled trials will, in practice, try to avoid any placebo effect.

Those who call themselves *healers,* and those involved in healing, act as a *catalyst* to expand consciousness for a wide range of individuals, employing common methods to provide key transformational input that will potentially enable such individuals to grow their awareness to such an extent that they can solve their real-life problems, solve and resolve their illness, and further their own needs and prosperity.

We all are walking and talking historical records of our cognitive couplings with our environment. It is this history of what we have been, which influences the way we interact with our environment in the future.

We each carry within us a unique notion of what constitutes 'good' health. Unfortunately, treating illness as *dysfunctional deviations* from so-called healthy individuals, or from the average of so-called healthy individuals, is about ensuring sameness, not uniqueness. To this extent, modern medicine is failing by adhering to a mechanical view of health instead of allowing the *unique* adaptation of each individual to the concept of health. A paradigmatic new approach to health would look at finding meaning in the patient's whole being and presenting symptoms. Organisms spend energy on internal organisation. With humans, this process is somewhat more complex. However, the patterns of practice – of how and on what the patient spends physical and mental energy – is either an adaptation, or a coping mechanism, the aetiology of which is the inability to sufficiently maintain a dissipative structure.

While the concept of placebo was introduced into medical research in an attempt to strengthen the methodology of testing the effects of *molecular medicine*, it actually brings our discourse back to consciousness studies. It also allows us to understand placebo and other related concepts such as metacognition, epigenetics, noetics, or bioenergetics as *self-regulating* activities by the human organism. Why? Because all these mechanisms allow the organism to react, on a molecular basis, on perceived environmental contingencies or the internal belief system. More to the point, all this can be achieved without having to first change the genetic blueprint, procreate, and wait it out for a generation or two. The adaptation to changing environments is almost immediate. The human organism has developed these mechanisms for the purpose of self-generation. This is perplexing, considering that mainstream medicine is predominantly concerned with randomised, controlled, trials-based, molecular and mechanical outcomes. Seeing this in context, research epistemologies may need to be revised in order to find a proper approach to the expanded view of nature and human nature.

What is colloquially termed an 'issue' is rather a strategy, a coping mechanism. Nobody knows how to run your own life better than you do. You are in charge, even though sometimes you may feel that you are not in charge at all. Whatever you believe about the world or yourself, whichever way you feel, whichever course you plot or action you take now, or will take in future, all this relates back to the situations that gave rise to such 'issues', and your cognition of them.

∞

Your life is a product of inside and outside forces and your response to those energies, thoughts, and emotional processes, infinitely nuanced as they reflect our individual personalities, our hopes, dreams, aspirations, disappointments, our feelings of anger, fear, resentment, our feelings of hopelessness, helplessness, loneliness, despair, contentment, and a plethora of other emotions and inner conditions. We create our realities on a daily basis, and should take much greater care in what we are bringing about. We need to face our own grandness and take a rather universal role and responsibility in a process of *cognitive health* by understanding our embeddedness and the reciprocity thereof of and about ourselves and the universe(s) we live in. This amounts to a conscious attempt to counteract entropy and to become all we can be.

> *We all live lives of partially realised greatness. We all experience tribulations, fear, anger, resentment, failure, despair, or sickness. And yet are we tasked to bring into alignment all that which we believe we are, or could be, and to remove such barriers towards self-realisation. Authenticity is an expression of the quality of resting within yourself by expanding your awareness about all of yourself.*

This, possibly, is our foremost commitment in life!

∞

NOOMON IV
∞
INNER TRUTH

When you look at yourself in the mirror, the following process occurs; light illuminates your body, is reflected in the mirror, and then enters your eyes through the lenses, creating an inverted image on your retina. The nerve signals reaching your brain then interpret it as whatever you are seeing. But *how do you see yourself?* Where does this image live? Your sensory organs carry the signals to the brain, and this is where the magic happens, within yourself. It is impossible to experience anything except within yourself. Whenever you touch an object in an apparently objective world outside of yourself, you are actually not touching it at all because the atoms in your skin actually repel the atoms of the object. On the atomic small scale, we never actually touch anything in this world. It is important to realise that everything that ever happened to you, good and bad, light and dark, pain and pleasure, joy and misery –the entire world – is sensed within yourself. Could this ever be a truly objective representation? Who has authority over the interpretation of all that data? Who adds awareness and cognition to such data and converts it into information?

Once you take ownership of cognition, it changes your entire experience of life; you understand it as being *mostly self-determined.* Even though the events around you might not be wholly determined by you, the experience of life is on this planet is, ultimately, determined by you. We have these internal representations of the world. It is a kind of simulation, a game we permanently run in the brain; it is this *simulated world* inside us that we act upon and react to. When our internal maps and our outside worlds, our *environments*, are not in sync and no longer congruent, we experience a *disconnect*. We label this disconnect a 'problem', 'something that doesn't make sense', a gut feeling of sorts.

> *How do we change the rules of the simulation game to avoid the experience of 'a problem'?*
>
> *Did somebody say 'simulation game'…?*
>
> *In an instant, this creates so many new questions.*

When we maintain that everything happens in the brain, and our bodies are just an extension to our brains, a vehicle to navigate the physical world, we could, in theory, imagine all the nerves as terminating on the surface of brain. But hold on, why do I feel these butterflies in my stomach, or the burden on my shoulders? Well yes, exactly. Why? What are emotions? Are they a reaction of the brain to the perceived congruence or incongruence of the internal map to the outside world? Would I experience or present an emotion if internal and external were in perfect harmony? Would you agree that, in the context of this discussion, emotions could be seen as positive or negative feedback loops? Those who engage in meditation regularly speak of 'being in tune with' or 'being at one with' the Universe, or the world around them.

> *In general, meditating generates an invaluable and fulfilling emotional response: peace!*

And so it seems that emotions allow us to be in the moment, they alert us to a – perhaps subconsciously – perceived congruence or incongruence that demands our attention, or at least our acknowledgement. Emotions allow us to be present, but to also find the motivation or 'energy' to act on a specific perception. The action you are taking is not on the external situation, but on your perception of it; it triggers you towards an emotional response of, say, anger or overflowing joy.

Can the internal simulation be aligned to the external 'reality', or, outrageously perhaps, vice versa? Can we go further and say the internal simulation *creates* external 'reality'? The external can influence the internal: I can set new goals, alter my model and shift my congruence by working on the exterior, to achieve that alignment and congruence again, through finding the exterior that reflects my subjective interior, and we could refer to the ensuing result as *balance*. This is an iterative cycle, a form of individualised learning and personal growth.

We see, hear, taste, touch, and smell. Through our senses, we internalise the outside world, we engage in simulations, we run what-if scenarios, we try to deduce an objective reality from subjective experiences. We establish belief systems about ourselves, our abilities, the world, God, the universe, my neighbour, nature: the list is almost endless. Because of this constant internal simulation game, the brain is used to predicting and analysing what happens next. We sometimes call it a *matrix* or something similar, and when we attempt to abandon our pattern recognition or creation abilities, we call it being *in the flow*. What we believe is true and valid in this world – norms, values, beliefs, views, thoughts, and so on – are really the iron bars of our cages. However, one always has the option of challenging one's own belief as much as one can challenge that of others!

Modern self-help techniques aim at breaking this simulation, to allow 'out of the box' thinking; to allow new impulses, leading to new views, to examine one's own views, to make our internal representations more objective and bring these into closer alignment with the outside world. Equally, cultural practices are often based on a certain theory of cognition, a way of dealing with emotions – life – and at times do not correspond with the simulation happening in the brain. This is sometimes referred to as a *belief system*, or a *paradigm*. Cultural practises are the belief systems, patterns, and ways of doing things that get imposed on individuals. This imposition disregards the simulation game going on in each one of us, and it requires people to comply with external standards that are, in general, institutionalised simulations in themselves.

Biologically, though, any incongruence means a *maladaptation* to the environment, and humans also use language to structurally connect to their environment. Why? Unlike most animals, humans can lie. We can easily say one thing, and do another, which means that, unlike a purely biological response, we can *create* maladaptation. We don't just talk, we talk to achieve *something*, to couple our internal representation or simulation to the outside world, to a *specific* outside world. These coupling processes are thus dialectic processes; sometimes we talk to *achieve* an input. In addition, people sometimes lie to themselves – the 'brain' says one thing but the 'heart' feels differently, and either one or neither is aligned with the external world. Ideally, the internal world should be fully integrated and authentic, but often it does not seem to be.

Updating your internal maps and reconciling them with the outside world requires a certain *flow* of energy. So what does free flow of energy have to do with internal mapping and congruence with the outside world? It has to do with the notion of 'dissipative structures'; all living organisms dissipate energy. Energy, in the form of food, water, information, words, etc. flow into the organism and gets converted, transformed, and used. It then flows out of the organism again as waste, as ideas, as creativity, as language, or as activity. Living organisms do that whilst at the same time keeping their internal organisation, structure and composition. Once that dissipative regulation fails, the organism will begin to fail and erode, just as rocks do. If pathways are not at least *similar* in terms of internal mapping and external world, the energy cannot flow. We absorb energy in vastly different forms; then we use it internally. When we talk about energies other than physical energies, we go back to the metaphor of the island in the ocean, surrounded by all kinds of energetic constellations that we convert into, for example, a belief about ourselves such as 'I am not good at maths', 'certain people who are xyz [replace xyz with any number of labels] are bad', or religious or philosophical concepts. At some stage, we develop internal maps that exemplify those beliefs, and we either allow dialogue and criticism from the outside to lead us to adjust these maps and return to less entropy, which in turn means better organisation and more congruence, or we attempt to find outside constellations that are congruent with our inner maps.

Having different pathways (or at least *some* internal mapping) which allow for different constellations of energies and configurations of life expressions, would explain why we all live on the same planet, but in sometimes vastly different worlds. Our internal representations are so vastly accurate and detailed, that we ascribe to them the label and status of *reality*. We act upon and react to this simulated world inside us constantly. We also constantly scan for congruence between the inner and the perceived outer world. Whenever the internal map and the outside world are no longer congruent, we experience an emotion, which, if it is negative, we call a *trigger*, an issue, or a problem.

OK, cool, but how do we avoid the trigger?

We often base our NOs, NOTs, MAYBEs, DON'Ts and NEVERs on an opinion about something, or an opinion by somebody about ourselves. Then we run with it as if that opinion about us is our reality, which it isn't. All this is based on the unequivocal understanding that 'consciousness' is the only viable quality of reality that could successfully serve as a container and a reason for all observable negentropic states of monistic reality. All reality frames and everything contained in them are a part of the same system of consciousness:

We are all connected!

Remember that there will always be enough reasons not to be, not to feel, and not to do! Amidst all the 'I have to...', the 'I need to...', the 'I cannot...', the 'I may not...' and all the other NOTs, MAYBEs, DON'Ts and NEVERs, you are really tasked with one goal only:

BE who you are.

As we will see in a later chapter, diversity is a primal principle of Creation. It is truly a human feature to take to monoculture, to standardise, to repress, outcast, shame, litigate, or condemn that, or those, who do not comply with those norms and values. It is a much discussed topic throughout human history, and human civilisations seem to go through phases of more or less acceptance of diversity. Understand that your island would be doomed if it consisted of only one thing. Accept that we humans are indeed capable of unifying diversity in an elaborate dance of alchemy; your island will feature dark and rough terrain as well as peaceful green pastures. Accepting either is a spiritual process of self-care!

On the inside you can set new goals, alter your model and shift your congruence, create the desired state. And then set out to find or create the outside that reflects the inside! This will result in a new balance, until a new iterative cycle of the simulation game begins. This is how we grow and learn. One of the secrets of life lies in 'self-acceptance', and from this comes 'forgiveness' for yourself and others; if you cannot accept yourself or forgive yourself, start off with something like 'Even though I cannot accept myself right now, I am ok' – work your way up from there.

∞

NOOMON V
∞
AMONGST MYSELF AND I

I s what we commonly refer to as reality nothing more than a mental construct? If it is a mental construct, can we as human beings choose what constitutes this reality we live in, and even choose our identity? And once we are into choosing, how much of our identity do we in fact choose? Are we a conglomeration of choices, whilst a plethora of external factors, e.g. family of origin, teachers, friends, social structures and social networks, media, as well as internal factors, seem to influence us and our decision-finding processes?

If among all those factors there are aspects we cannot choose, how did they come to form part of this construct we call identity?

Personality is a nonphysical entity, which means that we can only infer it from overt behaviour. The consistency of our interpretation of another's behaviour will eventually constitute a description of the other's personality. Every individual is in a conflicting state of satisfying inner, basic needs and justifying his or her actions in relation to the norms and values of society. In general, our *ego* will maintain the balance of reality between these two potentially conflicting, and at times, irreconcilable positions of pleasure and morality. While our drives and instincts mostly act on a subconscious level, the norms and values we experience are not necessarily experienced on a fully conscious level.

Yet what we refer to as being conscious, refers to the balancing efforts of our ego. When it comes to our forbidden drives, painful memories and feelings of guilt, which we love to repress in the dark realm of the subconscious, our thoughts and actions will be informed by them, even though this dark realm is an offshoot of the feelings, thoughts and experiences of our present awareness.

We colloquially call this consciousness.

The *healthy personality* is successfully able to satisfy its needs yet comply with the norms and values of society. This can be achieved without indulging in feelings of guilt or anxiety. This places an increased emphasis on the cognitive capabilities of the ego. Discernible stimuli within the environment have the power to exert an influence that moves an individual to react. These push and pull factors are able to either block or facilitate the expression of needs. Everybody has a different process of integrating these factors, and we refer to that difference as *individuality*.

Personality, then, is the characteristic behavioural pattern of balancing the interaction between internal needs and external push and pull factors. There is a tendency to seek a tension-free state, but there is also presumably a tendency to self-actualise, especially when it comes to the satisfaction of higher needs.

A number of components seem to be characteristic of a *healthy personality*, such as an extended sense of the self, a positive relation of the self to others, self-acceptance and emotional security, realism of perceptions and skills, insight, humour and the ability to self-objectify, and the attaining of a unifying philosophy of life. Ideally, we display a firm connection with reality, a readiness to express emotions, an ease of interaction with the environment, and realistic and honest perceptions of the self, others, and life as such.

Oh great… does that mean we are all unhealthy?

Phenomenology studies our subjective experiences, feelings and attitudes. Each individual lives in a world which is private to that individual, and where he or she can experience the central aspects of the 'I', the 'me', and the 'self'. This sense of self is basic and central to human functioning; the most basic strivings of the individual are directed towards the attainment, maintenance and actualisation of the self. In this process of *striving*, humans are proactive, rather than reactively being pushed and pulled.

The self-actualising tendency is the key concept in the unity of the individual, the motivation of the individual and its persistence over time; this is the process by which the individual reaches out for more competence. Self-actualisation is not merely concerned with the reduction of tension; it sometimes demands an increase in tension. As these processes are proactive, the increase in tension is not accompanied by negative outcomes; it is a dynamic flux which is the result of proactivity.

Why do different people attain different levels of self-actualisation? If self-actualisation is universal, why do people differ?

The answer lies in humanist phenomenology; we all live in our very own, subjective world. The individual will react to external stimuli according to the way he or she perceives that stimulus. The individual acts and reacts in line with his or her internal frame of reference, which encompasses everything and influences the way we see ourselves and how our concept of *Self* is constructed. Our Self is a differentiated part of the internal frame of reference, the phenomenological field. The Self is not responsible for guiding our behaviour. Instead, it is a feedback loop for reflections on topics such as one's existence, reality, or behaviour. The Self is the persistently valid corpus of the individual's evaluation of its own experiences. In general, when that Self is threatened, one tends to narrow one's phenomenological field in order not to perceive the threat, or one applies defence mechanisms such as *rationalisation* in order to minimise the perceived threat.

The notion of a 'healthy personality' is merely a tentative strategy to conceptualise and structure the many characteristics that we display in a way that gives rise to a certain degree of persistence and validity. The concept of the healthy personality implies a functionally better level of human existence. At root, this refers to the constructive adaptation of the organism to its environment. It doesn't really matter how this is accomplished as long as it promotes optimal interaction with the *outside*, and optimal integration of the *inside*.

Understandably, defining *identity* is fraught with daunting complexities. Uncountable defining characteristics and inner qualities meet myriad outer representations of our Self, making our identity more fluid than fixed at any given moment. Our identity is made up of those factors which we commonly attribute to our personality; our beliefs, our experiences, factors which get shaped and equally shape us along the way. Our Self, on the contrary, is defined by our cultural, religious, familiar environments, but include factors such as sexuality and gender.

∞

Personal growth is characterised by *lifelong learning*, by continually re-examining those factors which shaped us, and whether to abandon such information in lieu of new sensory input from the external world, or the evolution of inner states and emotions. All experiences – internal and external stimuli – are fundamentally assimilated in the mind and reorganised into an individual's reality. What constitutes *reality* is what we make of it.

Reality is a mere mental construct that one can rearrange and improve. Even a cursory glance at current self-help literature suggests that we have much more control and choice over what constitutes our identity than any preceding generation. As identity is driven by how we perceive our world, added knowledge about the world will enable us to exercise more control and more choice over what to include or exclude in our *identity* construct. To many, these processes of gaining knowledge about the world explicitly include empirical sciences as well as forms of faith, mysticism and intuition.

Identity seems to comprise those images we portray, the personal aspects we express, or the masks we wear, that many of us employ on a daily basis to project a certain persona. However, postmodern theories argue that creation of our identity is in fact subject less to conscious choice, and more to rather intricate, interactive patterns of action and reaction, of being shaped and guided by others while at the same time, shaping and guiding ourselves in response to what we perceive as acceptable, popular, trendy, or achievable. We are all embedded in networks of interaction, and those webs of dependency, co-dependency and interdependency force us to think and move in certain directions as we continually try to maintain our frame of reference. The postmodernist see identity as a collage, a tapestry of fragments of external influences, and the extent to which we choose our identity is a matter of debatable levels of consciousness. Awareness of these factors allows us to take responsibility, and being empowered by these liberating processes allow us to shift paradigm.

However, do we really *want* to choose our own identities? People are embedded in certain lifestyles that resemble movie scripts, narratives of self-identity that are transient and can be changed as self-perception changes. The way in which people react to the world is symptomatic of the 'external world versus internal world' dichotomy, the discussion about *man in the machine*; the question of whether we are just captains of a ship we call our body, sailing through the stormy waters that we call our world, giving rise to a rather defensive identity, the *I* versus the unknown and uncontrollable outside world.

Choosing one's identity nowadays seems more difficult than, say, a hundred years ago. Modern life is replete with contradicting forces, and given the discussion on the multi-layered experience of identity-finding, a high level of thought hygiene is required to discern between the pushing and pulling influences that nip away at our perceived hegemony, our freedom of choice. The mere terms 'freedom' and 'choice' immediately provoke greatly contrasting views, since 'identity' and 'self' have different meaning for people from all walks of life.

What does this mean?

It is all about making sense of the world we live in. The notion of 'choice' has a direct and empowering meaning to almost everybody. From this basis, identity-finding can achieve a higher, more inclusive quality than previously thought possible. Acknowledging the fact that reality is not as fixed and intransient as it seems allows people to take charge and change their lives, so that their lives become more in tune with their character traits. It allows them to adjust their identities and participate in their social, cultural and economic environments to experience increased levels of positive feedback, and ultimately, be closer to a unified epistemological worldview. But hang on: what is this state that we commonly call reality? Is it the sum of our sensory perceptions? What about those aspects and phenomena we cannot perceive with our senses, such as infrared light, radiation, nanoparticles, and atoms: are they real? And if they are, what is the meaning of the word 'reality'?

General psychology refers to the concept of *Self* as all those images *and* beliefs we entertain and maintain about ourselves. This self-image finds its genesis through accumulated memories that imprint on us since our childhood, and is obviously influenced to a great extent by important people in our lives. The concept of Self can thus be summarised as our *general perception of our behaviour, abilities, and character.* It is this image about ourselves that determines who we think we are as a person. It is important to understand that the image we have about ourselves may not necessarily be aligned with reality.

Although we have the exquisite ability to establish elaborate systems and concepts of *Self*, the design seems to be highly susceptible to *fear*. We all have our experiences and we all have a more or less pronounced yearning for certain, or just more, new experiences. The bandwidth is amazingly diverse, but can be conceptualised as a few categories. Two categories we strongly experience within ourselves are the things we are *good* at, and the things we are *not good* at. Let's call them our strengths and our fears. Our strengths are based on what we know to be true on the inside. Our fears are based on what we think to be true on the outside. *Can we really know what is true on the outside?* Not at all. But we start by making assumptions, and we internalise what is happening outside by developing a multitude of emotions, ranging from fear to heroism.

Humans just love to shriek away from pain and look for distractions to reduce or nullify it. This can and does take on the most bizarre and entertaining forms: substance abuse of all kinds, people-abuse of all sorts, self-abuse of all varieties, noises, distractions, self-restrictions, whatever the case may be.

Animals who have been subjected to traumatic experiences normally act out the shock. They will fight, run for hours, cry, shake, scream, exhibit abnormal breathing patterns, or hide. There is always some physical reaction involved. Humans have a huge frontal cortex which allows them to counterbalance the limbic brain. So we don't necessarily run, fly, scream, fight, jump or hide. Rather, we engage in non-physical activities such as mental, emotional, psychological or even philosophical responses, instead of working the trauma out of our system. This can take various, and sometimes in new layers of physical activities that seem unrelated to the initial trigger. For example, some may resort to cutting themselves with a razor blade, engage in drinking sprees, random acts of aggression, pleasure-seeking or danger-seeking behaviour; or engage in intellectualization, writing a book about the experience, overeating, substance-abuse, or developing health symptoms that are, at first sight, unrelated to the original traumatic event.

In a different context, this might be called 'culture', and often such activities become a culturally accepted way of dealing with such events. The most prominent examples include how men deal with war, and with those that come back from war, and also the celebrations and mechanisms of elevating so-called war heroes. In fact, many cultures around the world used to be matriarchal societies, until the society or nation was threatened in its values or functioning, came under attack, and then went to war. Patriarchy took over, and afterwards it remained stuck in that fight-or-flight state, instead of returning to its pre-war mode of operation. The universal occurrence of post-traumatic stress disorders, and our inability to deal with them successfully, has created an industry of institutionalised suffering. Up to today, almost all nations are *war machines at rest* rather than *peace machines at work*. Deplorably, almost none of our interventions fix the need of the organism to get rid of the trauma.

We should stop talking about people, or ourselves, as *having issues*. These are not issues but these are skills: the best adaptation the organism could come up with at the time. These skills can be extremely elaborate and intricate. At some stage, the organism was confronted with a situation or condition, within the body or outside, that brought forth a certain response. Once you allow the organism to react differently, it will – as a dissipative structure – restructure itself and develop different skills. With some guidance, those new skills will be based on less flawed assumptions about itself, and will allow it to base its life on its *strengths* instead of on its *fears*.

∞

Why not spend some time compiling a list of your fears? List them one by one, find a memory which addresses that fear, and look for the resulting belief about yourself from that memory. Write a possible alternative belief about yourself, had you had a different set

55

of coping skills back then. See whether you can find a memory that addresses that strength, possibly in a different context, and replace that memory of fear with the memory of strength.

Is the wooden table we sense as warm and solid – that *feels like wood* – really just that? Modern physics will tell us that the table consists of nothing more than a vast number of protons and neutrons, with electrons swirling around them, arranged and condensed in a certain pattern, and yet it appears to us in a totally different way. In a way, what we call reality is an epiphenomenon, an emergent property, of the structure and interaction of atoms and electrons. If this is the case, do we then see what we call *reality* as beyond our ability to perceive it?

Is there a reality *beyond* our perception? After we have built the best technology, the best microscopes, the best particle accelerators and spent ages researching the nature and extent of reality, will we then know what reality is? Once we have dissected the last component of an atom, will we have reached the end of reality, when there is nothing more to take apart? Will that then constitute all we know about reality, so that nothing we add or subtract from it will increase our knowledge about it? If there is an objective reality, independent of our observation of it, will we ever experience it as such? If human experience is subjective and subjective reality is a process whereby we filter and distort environmental input, could we remove human experience from the reality equation and let machines and devices do the measurements and analysis of observed, recorded, data? Will that then constitute a true reflection of reality? It gets even more complicated; does reality exist unless it is being observed, whether by humans or machines?

If you feel the wooden table now, and then get up and turn around, is the table still there? How can you ascertain that the table is in fact there without another observation? If one is to take quantum mechanics seriously, one must acknowledge the fact that the act of our observations pins down possible quantum states into observable and testable realities. One possible explanation could be that realities live in parallel, and we can tune into these at will, albeit not easily. Another explanation could be that the human mind is in fact able to create reality.

Quantum mechanics holds that matter, and thus reality, is simultaneously a particle and a wave. The act of observation is only possible if the particle loses its wave character and presents itself as a particle. Heisenberg's uncertainty principle calls this the 'collapse of the wave function'. The question arises whether the human mind is indeed capable of influencing 'hard' physics in such a way that the range of possibilities of the wave can be converted into an observable particle state. If yes, how could one devise a scientific procedure to test such an assumption repeatedly?

Is the wave function of matter weak enough to be influenced by thoughts, and if not, how strong is it really? What kind of energy is needed to collapse a wave function in order to get a physically tangible result?

The above very rudimentary explanation of quantum mechanics has various implications for metaphysical thought. For one, any given particle is, statistically, at many locations at the same time. This is referred to as the *wave function* and it describes the way a system can evolve. Until a measurement is introduced into the system which pins down the particle to a specific state, that particle exists in a multitude of locations. As deterministic as the physical world may appear to us, particles behave differently in quantum world. When you put a stone on the lawn outside, it will probably never shoot itself over the fence, but in the quantum world, an electron might do what is referred to as quantum tunnelling, and pass through an otherwise solid wall or change location all by itself. This sounds ridiculous, even spooky. And yet scientists are slowly discovering that quantum phenomena underlie physical world effects such as photosynthesis, smell, and possibly even consciousness.

Parapsychology has been testing such premises for decades, and yet we have very little scientifically valid data to corroborate their findings through testable and repeatable evidence, and many of their conjectures fall to Occam's razor. Many questions remain in quantifying the exact extent and nature of the human mind, cognition and the physical world; even more so in terms of quantum mechanics.

Yet human oral and written traditions repeatedly tell us of activities and effects which cannot be explained by Newtonian physics. The same goes for religion and mysticism; either such forms of knowledge about the world are an inherent function of the brain, or they are one of the strongest forms of self-deception ever devised by nature. In either case, the question arises as to why this is the case: is there a biological reason for this? Consider the following dialogue:-

Mary: *'I love John'*

Peter: *'What do you mean by "I love John"?'*

Mary: *'I mean, he is my husband, and I am devoted to him. I am content about this situation, and this constitutes for me the meaning of loving him.'*

Peter: *'Well, to me the meaning of love is defined by my understanding of self-identity. Love is a matter of accepting that the other person is part of the way I make sense of my immediate environment, and that the person is part of my identity.'*

In the example above, the notions and definitions of 'love' could not be further apart, though the two persons share the same language. In such a typical case of subjectivism we are faced with different value systems, one language, and two people. Is it actually possible to really understand what another person means when they say something?

What does it mean to say 'I know what you mean', or 'I understand what you are saying'?

Another striking example would be the discussion on abortion and the value of life. How do we define life? When does it start? Is abortion murder? What about the rights of the mother to create her identity, to create her own reality, to change the course of her life? The trap of subjectivism makes all of us live on islands, so that it is impossible to reach the other, and even by the definition of quantum mechanics, impossible to access the ultimate physical reality. The collective understanding of what is possible, or impossible, is referred to as a *paradigm*. Paradigms govern societies and countries, and are formed by the cumulative experiences of people who participate in the same cultural or sub-cultural environments.

The way we describe our world is an expression of the way we see our world, what we believe in, and what we contribute towards our culture, heritage, science, religion, art, and identity.

Admittedly, any such form of mediated knowledge gives some reason to presume our current worldview of *cause and reaction* is insufficient in explaining phenomena. Correlation between phenomena takes precedence over causation. The traditional scientific community will strongly disagree with this idea. However, does a new methodology and system of explaining the world beyond cause and reaction make sense? Does it allow for progress in areas where development has been stagnating? Will a new theory about our interaction with the world make us better human beings? Does it allow us to further our knowledge about the universe at large, the world and ourselves in particular, to a point where we apparently only have to think about change in order to achieve it?

If we consider that thought influences material reality, we should all be magicians. Are we? Can we create our day before we start to live it? Realities in different human societies look totally different. Scores of humans live under the most deplorable conditions across the globe despite quantum mechanics. The world does not seem to change just by thinking about it, and we still have to use muscle energy and fossil fuels to put one brick on top of another in order to build a house.

It would make much more sense not to postulate that we create and redesign the universe on a daily basis, that to a large extent we are in charge of and create our reactions to circumstances; or that we should allow ourselves a certain degree of openness to new stimuli; to reflect on one's current worldviews; to playfully embrace one's identity and, if needed, to replace stale and unsuitable concepts with more fitting, more helpful, more stimulating parameters.

Easier said than done, especially when all this seems like an unattainable luxury!

∞

Your island has many corners that might make you fearful. Not necessarily because monsters are lurking in the dark, but because you are more likely to be in totally unknown territory. Explore your island. Leave no stone unturned.

Once you start owning your space, you will start living more authentically. When we are tasked to include alternative epistemologies – ways and methods of knowing – in trying to understand the world and ourselves, we should rightly look to include knowledge gained by religion, mysticism and intuition in our paradigmatic theory of everything.

What if your relationship with yourself or others was based on a flawed assumption? Given your knowledge that everything you feel is on the inside, it's almost as if you are doing this to yourself, right? Would you agree that although something in your past only lasted for, say, fifteen seconds, it can reverberate like a bell within you for decades? Out of that may develop a fear which we relive or we try at all costs not to relive ever again. Whatever we do, we confirm that fear repeatedly, and we keep confirming the original incident or pain. We do this for as long as we keep resonating, and we prolong the ringing by entertaining those fears.

Fears are affirmations.

Make a note of any of these impossibilities that come to your mind. If they bother you, restrict or hurt you, try to open up to new possibilities; allow change. What do you have to lose? Understand that your belief and value systems not only guide you, they also protect you. Whether you need to change direction in life or make adjustments, at least be honest with yourself. This, more often than not, is an unpleasant experience. However, as you read this book, you will come to understand why honesty with yourself is absolutely necessary. As life progresses through different stages, several things change: the circumstances of life and living; the interpretation of reality and the way of reacting towards perceived stimuli; the nature, extent and direction of stressors; the cognitive and emotional coping resources of the individual; and lastly, physical and maturational changes in the individual. The interplay between factors determines the characteristic extent of the search for self-identity. Another function of self-identity is thereby achieved: stability and the ability to persist over time.

The concept of the *Self* helps to give direction and validity to the way the individual perceives and integrates stimuli from the environment.

Your island is thus not something that manifests overnight, only requiring some tweaks here and there. On the contrary, it is a lifelong project of *becoming*. You may be subject to, or prefer, a tumultuous process of shaping and redesigning. However, in the end, your life is an island amongst other islands, in a sheer endless sea of energy.

> *Your journey is a continuous spiritual search for self-identity.*
> *This is at least as dynamic as life itself.*

As much as early human development is dependent on a physical environment that nurtures the organism into growth, at some stage you may have developed sufficient self-reliance to lose that dependence; and you will be able to feel and think independently about the shape of your island. This is the stage where higher dimensions come into play: the experiences you have as an island do not define you, they just shape you. Although there is an intimate link between the shape of your island and its emotional quality, you are more than just that singular construct. You will come to realise that your island is just a physical manifestation of a *being* that is an expression of your consciousness, energy, and vibration. Whenever you are ready to do so, you will find the courage, the opportunity, and the strength to visit and revisit all your island treasures: its abysses, grottos, dark corners, jungles, pristine landscapes, beaches, cliffs, and mountain tops.

And ideally, you will come to realise that these are just experiences, and the question: *Who am I?* – will transcend those experiences, emotions, fears, angers, and loneliness and open up an inner world of great light, strength, and beauty.

You are the alchemist of your own life!

Whatever negative circumstances or constellations you find yourself in, understand that it is just a phase or stage. Allow this to pass, by letting go of the suffering. Open yourself up to learn from this. Learn whatever you can from the circumstances, and move on. Moving on does not mean leaving the circumstances, it just means that you are willing to change, that you are willing to let go of how things are in your mind. If you are bothered by the forest animals in your jungle, you cannot replace them with animals from the mountain areas. Everything in and about your island is in a cyclical relationship with its immediate, smaller and larger environments.

Most of these cycles are not accessible to our senses. We read about them in books, and they are given all kinds of fancy labels to show that they are *effects*, something extraordinary, potentially a runner-up to a *miracle*. Such effects show us that there are bigger cycles at play. Even though we can build mind-boggling skyscrapers, we are still embedded in nature, and our developments, small and large, as individuals and as a society, are natural processes.

Understand that your island is your sovereign land, no matter what others say or do. When you subscribe to getting to know your island and becoming intimately familiar with yourself, only good can come from your act of self-discovery. Whichever form or shape your island takes, there is a history of experiences, emotions, and thought processes behind it. Many of these will be below your awareness threshold, but you cannot really claim ignorance of them. Own them too, not just the beautiful beaches or breathtaking landscapes of your island; own it all.

Once you do, you will realise that there is even more to realise, to learn, to perceive, and to own. As you keep growing, you open yourself up to new possibilities and continue your journey. The Divine is literally waiting for you to start exploring, and by the time you have explored your inner worlds, you will turn your eyes even more *in*ward, and find *in* the island what you have been seeking *on* the island.

∞

NOOMON VI

∞

KNOWLEDGE MAKES THE
HEART GROW FONDER

Aren't you sick and tired of all the talk about energy and all this woo-woo stuff? Really now, can't we just go back to the good old material world and chill?

Yes, and no. In philosophical schools of thought, the basic dichotomy is termed *materialism* versus *idealism*; there either is a material outer world, or this outer world is a construct made up by each individual during the processes of consciousness. Immediately, another question raises its head: whether consciousness is just in our heads, or whether consciousness is also – or perhaps only – outside, while our brains act more like radio receivers for it. Are we perhaps living in a simulation with multiple takes on reality? Whichever flavour of woo-woo you choose to adopt, the 'other side' is often envisioned as being as complex and intricate as 'this side' of the veil. Sounds fascinating, but is there any truth in it?

The fact that we do not perceive our environment in the same manner as others do is an indication that truth is relative to the position of the individual. Concern over the essence and extent of culture is itself a cultural activity, and inasmuch as rationality is fundamental to our existence, so is the difference between individuals ultimately a cultural difference. Ultimately, many paths lead to similar insights, and although we are all travelling on subjective trajectories, we seem to traverse the same space. Bearing this relativism in mind, one could argue that cultural differences are differences not only in the perception of the world, but also in the employment of rationality.

As custom and tradition is absorbed through the process of socialisation, so are the laws of nature absorbed into individual or societal behaviour through a process: culture. At a very basic level every culture is parasitic upon the natural order and laws of nature. Naturally, this also entails a highly relativistic point of view, in that different strategies, at different cultural stages, hold equal 'truth'. The implication of this is that all models have been devised from a certain point of view: they embody a certain strategy, and they characterise a specific culture by exemplifying a certain perceived core problem. Thus, the *institutionalisation of the subjective world* equals an *establishing of the intersubjective world*, but only to the extent that it can function as a relief mechanism by substituting missing instincts. For example, the mechanism of the entire legal system and punishing criminals has its origin in 'purging' the community of illness similar to a shaman or medicine man doing this on a spiritual level. However, not all societies around the world practise this, even though every country has a legal system: in the Ubuntu tradition, the so-called perpetrator would sit in the middle of a circle of people, and they would talk good about that person and practise connection (instead of social isolation as Western societies do with their penal system).

On the other hand, one is tempted to see the abstraction of certain intersubjective experiences and their concentration in an institution as a softening of various differences: if a sufficiently large number of people perceive and experience the world in a certain way, so that one can institutionalise those experiences, and given that the process of institutionalisation is pure and objective, then that process is not only pragmatic, but also –presumably – close to reality. The employment of rationality does not mean that the fundamentals of logic are unevenly distributed across various cultural groupings, but rather that the diversity of life and the open-endedness of the world will tailor themselves to the need to apply rationality in a very pragmatic way.

What does this mean?

Firstly, take phenomenon X. This phenomenon can be explained in various ways, which could, and probably will, be differentiated by the *level of explanation*. Which level is to be chosen, meaning which explanation is to be accepted as *truth*, will be done according to Murphy's Law, or even Occam's Razor. Murphy's Law states that if a thing can go wrong, then it will go wrong. However, 'things' can only go wrong if they have the degrees of freedom to go wrong - the weaker the link, the more the likelihood that it will fail or go wrong. Occam's Razor can be reduced to four words: the simpler, the better...

Secondly, life is not only constituted by facts - the endeavour to investigate the world rationally will be restricted by the limitations of human logic when we confront concepts such as *love, truth, God,* or *pain.* Cultural differences do not rest in the individual as such, but rather in the processes of interaction that pattern and shape our lives. What we constitute reality to be determines our culture. Thus it is quite unimportant whether this is achieved by various *modes of thinking, institutional roles, systems of classification,* or by means of *power,* in the end these varied processes together constitute reality. Culture is neither an entity, nor is it an institution, but in every instance it confirms that we live in a man-made reality. Man-made, in this case, is used to denote everything that is perceived and experienced by the human being.

Where does this lead us?

Presumably to the understanding that the abstraction of common, yet individual characteristics or shared beliefs contributes to a higher-ordered system of interaction that constitutes what we refer to as culture. In this process, *institutionalisation, systems of classification* as well as *modes of thinking* play a role. In this way, a Christian society has a Christian culture, even though not everybody practises the Christian system of belief. In the same way, a 'Society of Lawyers against the Discrimination of AIDS-victims' is not a cultural group because it employs restrictions that allow only lawyers to be members of that group. As such, group coherence is not based on a dialectics of individual differences concerning their membership. Strangely enough, culture feeds off the diversity of individuals. One has to remember that a specific cultural grouping does not tell us what 'culture' is. One could, thus, differentiate between cultural groupings on the basis of different manifestations of culture, or one could do that on the basis of different interpretations of what is referred to as 'culture'.

The work of the philosopher Immanuel Kant, in his work *The Critique of Pure Reason,* laid the groundwork for empiricism, and he suggested that the world we perceive is a world we construe from empirical data; along the way. Others, especially Georg Wilhelm Friedrich

Hegel, in his work *The Phenomenology of Spirit*, adopted a different position by maintaining that the relationship between the human mind and the universe is very much dialectical in nature, that our existence is essentially a constant process of defining a thesis, reacting with an antithesis and construing a synthesis. To the extent that every synthesis can be a new thesis or, an antithesis, human knowledge will progressively reset until it reaches the ultimate – the *Absolute Idea* – which is at the very heart of Hegel's metaphysical system of Absolute Idealism.

To the extent to which a hypothesis (thesis) will *map* a phenomenon of the real world, our experience will never be more than a mere source of probability. However non-*realistic* this probability might be, it still constitutes reality, and science, for that matter, always rests on the latest iteration of falsification. According to Hegel, this means that as long as we assert something by stating a thesis, and at the same time negate it by stating the antithesis, we will conclude with a synthesis that which will always be within the phenomenological field of the human mind. Hegel maintained that anything we think of can exist; anything outside our phenomenological field would be totally inaccessible to us.

It is important to note that the progressive restatement of human knowledge resembles a hierarchy of reality and truth. Where Kant would have separated *appearance* and *reality* into opposites, Hegel maintains that the two are separated by a matter of degrees, thereby applying the principle of the *unity of thought*. The separation between the object and the thought is very much a separation within the thought itself. This means that all appearances that we take to be *reality* are in fact a separation (of degree) within the overall *Absolute Idea*. Put differently, where there is conscious experience, there also is an object of experience. In the same way, where there is an object of consciousness, there must also be a state of consciousness for which there is an object. There is thus always an object-in-someone's-consciousness, and equally there is only a situation-in-someone's-consciousness. Never will there be an object only or situation only.

Hegel's *unity of thought* introduces another important aspect: *truth and falsity*. Truth and falsity are closely connected with the principle of progression towards *the Absolute*, a process which is unstoppable and that underlies the unity of the system of ideas. Truth is not seen as mere correspondence, but rather as an internal correspondence between being and thought. As every assertion, every negation, every appearance is borne out of *the Absolute*, the very criterion for the instance's truth is immanent in the unity of thought or, put differently, internal to the instance, irrespective of whether it is an assertion, a negation or just an appearance which we take to be the reality. Hegel's theory of truth has important implications for philosophy. Firstly, reality is self-contained; there is no dichotomy between appearance and reality. Reality is the very first and the very last instance to which any form of truth or falsity can and must be related. This is so, because there is no other reality than that which is contained in the unity of thought.

During Hegel's lifetime (1770-1831), philosophy was seen as the umbrella for other sciences rather than as its foundation, as it is regarded today. On the other hand, one has to bear in mind that, according to Hegel, a human being is not a singular being superseded by the rest of creation, untouched and untainted by that which he is to dominate. This view is more reminiscent of previous philosophical landmarks: Descartes (1596-1650) posing the anguished choice of being or non-being, or Kant (1724-1804) proposing the case for being utterly rational and categorically imperative.

It was Hegel who inserted the notion of all individuals being tied together in one and the same life-world, with as many options to act on as there are individuals who can relate themselves to the objects in the environment. This kind of systems thinking laid the foundation for later generations of everything from systems theory to chaos theory, and one could safely say that Hegel's system has constructively worked against Kant by arguing that human reason can indeed provide certain principles of explanation or schemes of rationalising which reach beyond the Kantian limits of human rational ability. In addition, Hegel made his system very rational in providing only one – albeit religious in character – overall principle; the unity of thought and the authenticity of reality, a notion which rather infuriated existentialists.

At its core, the origins of American New Age thought can be found in ancient Indian philosophy, or even in the world of Plato in ancient Greece. The resurgence of European philosophy advanced with the advent of Goethe and Hegel, amongst others. This had considerable influence on the *American Transcendentalism* of Emerson (1803-1882) and the *New Thought* of Quimby (1802-1866). Other authors, such as Hill, and Atkinson, had a formative influence on American New Age thought, which in the second half of the twentieth century spread to Europe and found willing participants, proponents, and scholars across the entire Western World. It spawned an enormous number of esoteric movements, with some reaching even to the East. Inasmuch as the American Spiritualist Movement is based on a spawning of the works of preceding thinkers and proponents with a bewildering proliferation of 'secret knowledge' and creating 'secret societies', the content is largely based on Hegelian philosophy.

∞

We have to give quantum physics the credit for steering the discussion about energy in a new direction. It took decades for physicists to wrap their heads around the perplexing and counter-intuitive measurements and consequences of quantum physics. At the heart of this conundrum lies the realisation that there is no such thing as the material world as we had come to understand it over the past millennia. Yes, the table we are touching feels solid indeed, but looking at the subatomic structures of the table, there are atomic nuclei, and electrons. Looking deeper, we see smaller particles, but essentially these are nothing more than statistically significant distributions of energy. Why such energies aggregate and create something we call an atom, a molecule, a protein, a table, a star, or a universe is a major point of discussion. It was similarly found that the Higgs boson flips the normal curve statistical distribution into something we call *mass*, and for this reason it is often referred to as the *God particle*. Mass is the building block of a materialist universe. Yet we find that as much as light is material, it does not respond to gravity like a falling apple does, but takes up a special case of mass being able to move at extraordinary speeds. This had implications for seeing the universe, or material reality, as mechanical, as we had come to believe.

What we take away from the realm of physics is twofold.

All of reality is energy,

and

All energy vibrates.

The consequences of this are disastrous for our mechanistic view of reality, because in as much as we have successfully tested and applied mechanical principles to the movement and interaction of 'objects' such as stars, gears, falling apples, or flying projectiles, and distilled these observations into what we call natural laws or laws of physics, quantum physics shows us that everything is more akin to energy and less to objects. Also, if everything is energy, why does everything vibrate, where does that oscillation, that vibration, come from? What is driving this?

The acknowledgement that everything is energy and vibrates has important consequences for energy healing. What does it actually mean when one needs to 'change one's vibration', to 'vibrate at higher frequencies'? How do we go about achieving this, and, *is it true?*

Does truth actually matter, if everything is consciousness?

∞

You have barely settled on your island, and barely come to terms with the vast tapestry of shadows and the character of the various areas and crevices of your island, and now this. Quantum physics is telling you that none of this is actually true, and yet it is. This is ridiculous, right? Do I exist, or don't I? Do I have a body or not? Am I hallucinating reality? All this can be very confusing, and you might be losing your grip on what you thought is a pretty much reconciled physical reality. However, there is a line of thinking and inquiry into the nature of reality that reaches back into antiquity and seems to have its first documented roots in the Vedic writings of India. It is quite possible that this system of thought is even older. Who knows for sure, right? It would be negligent to dismiss this ancient philosophy, which paints a totally different picture about the nature of reality than what established Western cultural trajectories teach us, while at the same time refusing to engage in serious scientific discourse on alternatives to the Western model of reality.

To this day, the topics of energy, energy field, vibration, frequency, consciousness, and even alternative accounts of the origin of life, creation, humanity, and many more areas of interest are met with ridicule, shame, dismay, religious fervour, dogma, refusal, or even punishment and incarceration.

And yet - as much as we are used to a so-called physical reality - we switch language as soon as we talk about our feelings, emotions, or inner worlds. Suddenly we 'feel' pain, sorrow and joy; we 'feel' our 'energy' draining away or invigorating us; we 'feel' the 'knot' or the 'butterflies' in our stomachs. None of us talks about nanograms of chemicals whizzing around and attaching to receptors, of sugar levels plummeting or blood pressure stretching our capillaries. All this we do automatically, without even considering that the way we measure and account for the outside world is totally different than what we do for our internal world. Instead, we postulate a duality of body and mind, we find philosophical differences between the quality of matter and the quality of emotions or thoughts, and perhaps, as in the picture of you seeing yourself as an island, there is no difference at all.

> *All of reality is of the same substance, which is no substance at all. No matter how deep we look, everything seems to point to a higher order reality and First Cause. And yet there are millions of people who live very successfully without resorting to any form of divinity.*

Once you become aware of and have experiences of the concept of *better, fuller, richer, more colourful*, or being *true to yourself*, this cannot be undone. You cannot undo the effects of knowledge gained from self-discovery. We all end up with various viewpoints for different reasons, and we all walk different paths through life. We are not necessarily any wiser about the concerns of the world around us, but we all know ourselves a little bit better.

To some of us this might be excruciatingly scary, or it might just be an awesome joyride. Yet, once you take ownership of your emotions, your thoughts, your ideas, your pains and your joys, you begin owning your life, and you begin knowing better how to navigate your life. This doesn't mean you now suddenly have to be, or *may* be, irresponsible and happy-go-lucky. It means that you are beginning to be more true to yourself, and that just may put you on a different path through life, irrespective of your age and experience! There are many things in life that we just *don't know*, and there are many things we may have no interest in finding out either.

There is freedom in saying 'I don't know.' When we admit that we don't know something, we can then open ourselves up to the opportunity to learn. And this has tremendous potential to heal!

So then, let us return to your island. Parts of your island will have sheer drops, or cliffs that are subjected to the full force of the tides. These are areas of brute force. Other areas of your island will have beaches; same water, same island, but the mood here is different. Here, you will find more harmony and less brute force. In both scenarios, the force and its effects coexist. There might be abrasive action from water to some degree on the harmonious beaches, but its effects on the cliffs, its shaping of the landscape, is much more dramatic. Here, you start understanding the concept of give and take, you start observing cycles, chaos and the abrasive pain that creates beauty in the process of alignment. Remember though, in this picture aligning your island *means* aligning your *Self*.

Understand that behind everything on your island, whether cliffs, beaches, inhospitable jungles, mountains, crevices, plains or dark grottos, there operates a more or less limiting belief about yourself that is bigger than the island, possibly, but not exclusively, spiritual in origin and nature.

What you see as living your life is akin a reconnaissance mission to find those beliefs about yourself, and everything else, that stand between you, yourself, and the Divine.

Once you find these limiting beliefs, you will be able to let them go - once you are ready to let them go. It does not matter whether these beliefs hurt you in the process of living, or whether they allow you to prosper and excel. What is important is that you gain as much knowledge about yourself as you possibly can. Only then will you become increasingly unaffected by the waters around you.

∞

NOOMON VII

∞

REINCARNATION AND THE TRANSFER OF KNOWLEDGE

In a nod towards Teilhard de Chardin (1881-1955) and his *Phenomenon of Man*, a number of emergence theorists suggested that although the universe is made of matter, it is rather evolving. While the matter in the universe is falling into entropy, ultimately life and consciousness may be able to escape this fate by becoming forms of information which are material-independent, i.e. patterns of organisation, and entering into hyperspace or other dimensions. 'Mind' is postulated as something which is emerging and may possibly leave its material substrate. This connects to the notion of reincarnation; continued cycles of reincarnation could eventually lead to a life independent of a physical body, allowing us to escape from entropy.

Mysticism has its roots in the premise that there seems to be purpose in the universe, that the universe seems optimised for the emergence of conscious observers. However, this premise leans toward pantheism, implying that this is ultimately part of the universe's 'plan' to save itself from entropy by necessitating and facilitating the emergence of reproductive (self-replicating), reflexive (self-organising), and then reflective (self-aware) systems that can preserve or even create order.

Unlike the reductionist tendencies of traditional science, the emergence of synthetic viewpoints in science – chaos and catastrophe theory, systems theory, cybernetics, holism, ecology, and so on – suggests a trend towards a fundamental awareness of the more subtle aspects of matter, tending towards synthesis and holism. Researchers and thinkers such as Giordano Bruno (1548-1600), Robert Boyle (1627-1691), and Isaac Newton (1643-1727), are grounded in Gnostic traditions that were critical of organised religion of their days, but not necessarily or similarly hostile toward spirituality.

This Gnostic viewpoint of knowledge of the universe leading to self-knowledge - and thus enlightenment - is at the basis of the well-known *as above, so below*. Only when we know all aspects of the world do we come to know our true selves. To this extent, the overarching process of bringing forth worlds is that *knowing is doing*. The process of liberating the Self is but just a first step in the grander process of universal liberation. When we refuse to consider new revelations, when we stay focused only on the past, when we eschew technology and artifice, will this lead to entropy, isolation, and death, physical and spiritual.

Reincarnation as a theory is widespread in the East, with its epicentre in India and branching out to countries that have adopted Buddhist or Hindu faiths. As a theory, it is closely linked to the concept of karma, in that good actions in one life are rewarded in subsequent lives, while bad actions lead to suffering in subsequent lives. The concept is therefore closely linked to a certain view of morality. In some forms of Buddhism, there is a strong emphasis on karma as part of teachings on morality, which contrasts to the Buddha's reluctance to give any emphasis to individual reincarnation; that is, to any speculation about an individual's previous existences. Reincarnation as a theory is accepted by the peoples of the Hindu, Buddhist, and Jain areas of the East, but for most it probably remains a theory on the same level as Darwin's evolutionary theories do for the peoples of the Western worlds.

Various texts from Eastern philosophical and esoteric traditions deal quite specifically with reincarnation; the Tibetan Book of the Dead being a unique example. The Tibetan Book of the Dead prescribes a series of recitations at the deathbed of an individual to help him or her deal with the in-between stage; to see the increasingly physical 'apparitions' in their descent to rebirth as projections; to resist the descent by clinging to the purity of the earliest phase; to resist the last phase, that of apparitions of copulating couples; and finally, if unable to resist the pull of sexual imagery, to remain as pure in thought as possible to secure a favourable birth.

While reincarnation has no official place in the three major religions of the west, there is a long history of the subject in the West, starting with Pythagoras, through Plato, to Jung, Papus, Rudolf Steiner, and Edgar Cayce in more recent times. Other Western writers on reincarnation include Swedenborg, Jacob Boehme, Madame Blavatsky, Annie Besant, and Alice Bailey. Steiner perhaps attempted the most public elucidation of the subject, while Cayce was a rather reluctant convert to the belief in reincarnation. Reincarnation is more clearly part of esoteric or occult traditions in the West, and probably attracts a more polarised response of acceptance or rejection than in the East.

To the public, Carl Jung (1875-1961) presented a dismissive view of reincarnation, though he may or may not have had other thoughts in private. However, in his work *Memories, Dreams, Reflections* there are numerous passages that are reminiscent of past-life recall, particularly where he muses on why some people who cross one's path stand out and others do not. Jung is not in favour of the Oriental concept of reincarnation, but later debates the issue in a more open way. Jung's comments can be taken to support any number of ideas, including: reincarnation, his own theory of the collective unconscious, and the tradition of the *Akashic Records*, in which everything that has ever happened and will ever happen is already written down. His conclusion, however, is that he cannot tell whether the karma that he lives is the outcome of his past lives or rather his ancestors, but he suspects that if he had lived in previous centuries he was now born to answer unanswered questions. In his psychological commentary on the Tibetan Book of the Dead, Jung decides more definitely against the continuation of a personal history, favouring the archetypal or ancestral theory.

The objections to the theory of reincarnation are interesting to consider. In both East and West, sceptics point to mechanistic problems, the main one of which is that the population is growing, so where do the new 'souls' come from? The more materialistic Western mind, with its emphasis on scientific knowledge, also objects to the persistence of memory and personality implied by reincarnation: memories and personality are a function of the brain, so when the brain dies they disappear.

The Buddha's objection is more significant for mysticism: it is not relevant or helpful to speculate on the subject. Silence of the mind is the path (or goal); consciousness is more important than its contents, particularly memories, whether of this life or any other. Western objections, other than the 'scientific', are less clearly articulated, and more open to speculation. The Western concept of the individual, or the primacy of individuality, sits uneasily with the concept that one could have been someone else, particularly someone with opposing views and attitudes to those one currently holds, and relates to a certain rigidity of personality.

However, one could reinterpret the concept of reincarnation differently. For instance, reincarnation could be seen as an information-saving mechanism within a larger dissipative structure, similar to our DNA being preserved and passed on to our offspring in our embodied, physical, dissipative structure. Reincarnation would thus resemble a metaphysical evolutionary strategy.

But why would there be an evolutionary benefit to this?

One reason could be the development towards the *Higher Universal Mind*, the universal development of conscious life in particular and all creation in general towards what was elsewhere termed the *Omega Point* by de Chardin. Alternatively, reincarnation could be interpreted as a phenomenon based on information only, without reference to karmic or purgatorial principles. Taking this approach, there would be no bad person, or good person, and there would be no sin or punishment.

However, there would be good information, and bad information. Bad information would foster bad feelings and bad behaviour such as hatred or mistrust. Good information, such as enlightenment by the Higher Self, would foster good feelings and good behaviour. Good information would encourage learning and adaptation within an open system, counteracting entropy and allowing for a dissipative exchange of energy and development. Bad information would encourage closed systems, entropy, pollution and non-disclosure.

As a theory, reincarnation relates to the concept of karma: good actions in one life are 'rewarded' in subsequent lives, while bad actions lead to suffering in subsequent lives. The concept is therefore closely linked to a certain view of morality. It also leads to the inexplicable – to Western mindsets – tolerance of suffering, people living in abhorrent poverty with a smile on their faces.

However, if we interpret karma in terms of information theory, the concept loses its fatalist dimension. Karma does not encourage dissipative systems. Staying within the analogy to closed entropic systems, karma is the residual energy which the system can no longer use for further action. This resembles the alchemical concept of *terra damnata*, except that earth is not damned. Karma is not a burden, not a curse, not hell, not damnation. It acts like a disposition, degenerating and wearing down a system which could otherwise flourish as an open system. You can battle it, wing it, celebrate it, up to you - until you grow your consciousness.

It is also possible to postulate reincarnation as an emergent property or pattern of interaction between highly complex systems. The discussion on self-generating living systems allows us to postulate reincarnation as a self-generating network pattern, and suggest that reincarnation is a result of interaction with others and the environment in such a way that, specifically, positive feedback loops stimulate the system to such an extent that bifurcation happens.

However, is reincarnation a process of cognition? Does reincarnation move along the lines of memory, similar to DNA being a biological memory system? Is reincarnation a structural coupling of the individual to its environment? If so, which environment, and more so, who, or what, is coupling to what – soul-to-universe, or soul-to-soul, or soul-to-body? Could karma be the result of a systemic function instead of an individual complexity? And does bifurcation apply to reincarnation similarly to the way it applies to complex biological systems? Does a system need to be embodied in order to behave like, or similar to, a physical system we are observing? When we look at the complexity of ant behaviour, traffic, weather, sand piles, societal systems, can we in all instances talk of embodiment?

The concept of reincarnation is of particular interest in relation to the concepts of *information* and *entropy*, as it refers to a principle or a mechanism of 'recycling' of information in the context of the existence of human beings within the framework of this universe. The combination of entropy and information theory within a bigger framework of complexity theory allows for a new interpretation of reincarnation. Consequently, the question asked here is whether recycling, or the re-introduction and re-use of information and energy (soul) is a universal strategy to counteract entropy.

Alternatively, after dismissing reincarnation as the transformation of the psyche through the relationship between the ego and the contents of the unconscious, including the collective unconscious, the theory of dissipative structures and complexity theory allows for a reinterpretation of consciousness, reincarnation, information, mind and spirit as emergent phenomena; epiphenomena which have no metaphysical relationship to the biological substrate that harbours those processes. This implies that the process of reincarnation is a process of lowering entropy, a process of raising the information content or the information quality within the higher order system.

Spiritual growth is thus a defining principle in understanding reincarnation, information, and entropy within a framework of complex systems and how non-linear systems operate, interact and relate to each other, whether in a hierarchy of higher-order systems or not. Spiritual growth is a mechanism to lower entropy, to raise levels of consciousness, to positively stimulate a system into bifurcation. The question then arises: bifurcate into what? Closed systems will bifurcate into a state of higher equilibrium, open systems will bifurcate into more diversified iterations, or into a more specialised iteration. Presupposing that spiritual growth equals a bifurcation into a more specialised iteration requires a specific notion of what growth means, and whether specialisation is good information or bad information.

When we equate DNA to a biological preservation mechanism, and reincarnation to a spiritual preservation mechanism, we still need to figure out where the spiritual information resides. DNA creates proteins, and those proteins are folded and repackaged, create enzymes, and are used in all kinds of mechanisms, cycles, and systems. As such, DNA is just data. Is that true? There is no information in DNA other than instructions for RNA to produce proteins. We thus have two engines that drive our development and our existence – the first is the biological, the human-animal part. The other is the spiritual one, the growth towards the Divine. The biological engine has an awesome memory preservation mechanism we call DNA, but the spiritual one is seemingly lacking. However, various teachings have found various answers to this question.

Reincarnation demands that we respond to and consistently live with the call of the Divine Creative that we are; it demands that we act as autopoietic systems, open and ready to embrace this life, and thus demands a tremendous degree of self-responsibility, self-integrity, and inner freedom. Self-responsibility is the ability to respond to the summons of our Higher Self to attempt the path of our singular cosmic destiny; self-integrity is the ability to live our lives in a manner that is consistent with this summons and with the creative vision of ourselves. Metaphysical freedom demands that we are possessed of inner authority and authorship, while remaining independent of all forms of external authority in the matter of thinking and knowing. Enacting such evolutionary principles and responsibilities, by creating order, bestowing meaning, and allowing a metaphysical autopoietic dialogue within oneself and with one's environment, is the teleological essence of metaphysics.

The creative vision that we are is the singular yet universal call of the Universal Mind, that we are indeed capable of accessing the unknown within us and our cognitive context. As in the case of a closed physical system within which entropy continuously increases, a person who is closed to the unknown is also closed to the possibility of spiritual development, which is the conscious process of creating an increasingly higher order or greater syntropy within, ceaselessly dissipating entropy. In the spiritual context, order or self-organisation is synonymous with wholeness. Therefore, spiritual development is the attainment of increasingly greater wholeness of being, of increasingly more holistic unfolding of the Higher Self. In the context of entropy and negentropy, spiritual awakening is an *order-generating process*. Self-responsibility and self-integrity are the essential keys that unlock the opening for this syntropic process of spiritual development and awakening.

Dear Island, in the vast endless ocean, do you trust your instincts, your capacity for sound judgement, the strength to assess life properly, or your own set of beliefs and knowledge? If you have something big coming up, would it help trying to change your focus to being okay with the decision you are about to make?

Perhaps you need to open up to possibilities of finding a *different* solution, or finding a *different* decision. Perhaps you are guided too much by fear, or resentment, or any other emotion that prevents you from being fully present in the moment? Think about the sheer cliffs on one coast of your island; you would not go there confidently because you might be afraid of heights, or perhaps it is too eerie, too dangerous, too forbidden? If you cannot process the issue cognitively, pass it on to your subconscious, and whatever comes up, whatever it is to be, you will still be okay with it.

One lesson we need to learn is to *trust ourselves*. If we don't, we will forever be looking to others to prove our own merit to ourselves, and still never be satisfied. We will always be asking others what to do, and at the same time resent their help.

> *Trust in yourself starts with being okay with the consequences of your decisions.*

We overwhelmingly reduce our experience to a handful of sounds we call words. This is, no doubt, useful or even necessary for living in (modern) society. But it's all too easy to lose touch with the reality these grunts aim to describe. We label emotions too. We quest after something called *happiness*, thinking there must be a readable formula for *joy*. But at the core, don't we simply crave pleasant feelings? These moods, of course, can't be talked about with any accuracy but only felt.

Often, we think too much, and these thoughts are constrained by language. We even think about thinking (like right now).

It may even be necessary to just let go of words for a moment in order to taste reality, whatever that is.

Even if life doesn't feel awesome to you right now, how about some mindful meditation and enjoying the bliss of being alive, something like:

> *'Even though life is really tough at the moment, perhaps I could allow myself to just enjoy this moment.'*

∞

Your first step is always to acknowledge where you are, allow the lesson to happen and allow yourself to be taught, even though this might be painful.

Don't let anything come between you and yourself. Your perception of *Self*, and your being an island in the ocean, need to be as much aligned as possible. There will always be reasons why this shouldn't be the case, or perhaps you are actively prevented or prohibited from being *at one with yourself*. Maintain that personal movement towards intimacy with yourself; this is where your Higher Self is waiting for you.

Practise to be *reflective*, to be self-aware. This self-awareness will foster the necessary self-responsibility for spiritual growth. Understand that your existence as an island has nothing to do with the opinion of anyone else in this universe about you. Cover as much ground on your island as possible. Identify with as many facets of your island as possible, and bring all that into your awareness. However, this is only the first level of making sense of it all.

Practise to be *reflexive*, to self-organise. You will need to integrate your acquired knowledge into the way you relate and integrate with your environment(s). What are you about to do with all this knowledge about yourself, about every little nook and cranny of your island? What is there to gain from all this? For some, this is burdensome. Either they are too busy with their lives, making ends meet, struggling with all kinds of push and pull factors; or it is just too painful to get more insight into your *Self* as an island. Either way, it just is too much, too overwhelming. Why burden an otherwise busy mind with even more stuff to ponder?

> *The only knowledge you can know you have for sure, is about yourself. The rest is really just hearsay!*

87

Objective reality does not exist, and those machines we are building, the sciences we are establishing, the so-called facts we are assembling, do not relay knowledge about the true nature of everything, but only how it appears to us or to our instruments. At some stage of your self-organisation you will realise that everything you learn about the world are the characteristics and qualities of that which we call 'reality'. It is an interpretation of some sort. Be aware of this. Challenge what you know. And challenge the ways and methods you employ to obtain that knowledge.

Practise to be *responsive*, to self-create. Create order, bestow meaning, yet recognise that all order is arbitrary, and that paradigms, rules, and order, can be changed without prior notice. You are entitled to change direction in mid-air. That doesn't make you unreliable, it just means that you integrate knowledge differently, and that you choose to self-create based on integrating what you learn about yourself.

> *Allow yourself to change, yet maintain integrity. Allow yourself integrity, yet change.*

Know that trying to 'stay the same' despite a changing environment actually leads to loss of integration, loss of information, loss of self-authority.

∞

NOOMON VIII

∞

HEALING AND THE SHIFTING
OF GOALPOSTS

Philosophical thinking in the West over the past 2,000 years has significantly shaped our thinking about emotions, and about the ego. The works of Sigmund Freud on the id, the ego, and the superego have perhaps limited our degree of freedom for personal expression. The ego is something that is judged harshly in Western societies. In fact, it is in direct opposition to altruism and social responsibility programmes of all kinds.

The notion that a healthy expression of *Self* is essential to mental health is almost a taboo subject in many societies. We have more or less flattering names and labels for such individuals: go-getters, egocentrics, or egomaniacs, people who are out for instant gratification, ego-trips, over-the-top, exhibiting small man syndrome, narcissistic behaviour, and many others. We enlist art therapy, music therapy, imago therapy, cognitive behaviour therapy, psychodynamic therapy, Gestalt therapy, group therapy, electrotherapy, and many other forms of therapy or interventions to corral the ego, to allow its expression in more 'socially acceptable' ways. And yet, the ego is a necessary antecedent for *self-care*.

In its own time, life provides you with sufficient answers. You could access these answers through prayer, meditation, tapping, practising art or solitude, and many other forms of contemplation.

> *'Even though I do not understand why things are the way they are, I trust this is leading me to somewhere good.'*

Throughout life, we keep creating and co-creating as we are shaped and formed. It never stops, and we never seem to be able to escape this. Even in failing, there really is no failing; provided that you understand the lesson.

> *'Who would I be if I were to allow my life to change, or this person to change, or some or other circumstance to readily transform?'*

Anne is married to Peter. Peter is working in a big insurance company and had a rather superficial affair with his secretary. Anne found out and was devastated. She tried to put it all behind her, but the memories live on and the following conversation with a friend ensues:

Anne: Just went into my archived WhatsApp messages and came across Susan's message where she confessed to me that she and Peter were physical and kissed a few times, but never slept together.

Garreth: Nothing new there, we knew that...

Anne: I wonder if the anger and hurt attached to that ever goes away. Life and its doughnuts... lol

Garreth: Sit for a moment, and leave your body. Imagine you are the *Universe*. Look at things from a bird's eye view, and at the same time, be impartial and positive about every one of the people you see down there...

How would you interpret Peter's actions with Susan?

And how would you see this individual called Anne, sitting somewhere and feeling angry, and hurt, and rejected, and unloved, and ignored, and all the other emotions she is coming up with just to justify that she is worthless?

What would you say, if you took the dialectic position of 'the Universe', about Peter, and about Susan, and about Anne...?

Anne: My reply would be something like: 'You are all lost. It's your responsibility to find your way. Start working.'

Garreth: So, what made them lost?

Anne: They felt unfulfilled in their situations. Frustrated.

Garreth: Frustrated, unfulfilled, OK. So why did they choose the way they chose? Why didn't they choose a totally different path?

           How would you live, how or who would you be, if every person you met, in whichever form or way, was a representation of The Divine? And every single time, you have the option to reach out, or withdraw. The emotions you feel actually help you to be 'in the moment', but what are you prepared to *create* in every one of those instances...?

Anne: Love and upliftment. The answer comes naturally but action is a bit more difficult.

Garreth: OK, so your body generates this emotion, let's give it a name: *hurt, with a touch of disbelief and anger*. This emotion is present, right now, after reading Susan's message. OK, so now you are present, right? Your emotions have your full attention. And now, create!

           The question is: what are you going to create? *The Divine* gave you this power; what are you going to do with it?

Anne: It's hard to say; understanding, flowing from love. Releasing her after she has been uplifted.

Garreth: Another thing *The Divine* gave you: you are free to choose what you want to create, even if you decide to create negativity.

93

Anne: OK, I want to kick her ass. Bitch!

Garreth: Sure, OK; and what are you creating here?

Anne: And he is a prick! Creating hate here!

Garreth: And how does this hate-creating make you feel?

Anne: It doesn't feel right, instinctively.

Garreth: OK, but you are still free to do it.

Anne: I am. I need to feel neutral! I can't feel positive about it because I am resisting that, and feeling negative feels bad.

Garreth: You do feel neutral? What are you creating whenever you feel neutral?

Anne: Peace...? Indifference.

Garreth: Is peace the outflow of neutral? What about forgiveness? Is that an outflow of neutral?

Anne: Maybe indifference is... If you forgive does it mean you trust again?

Garreth: When you are indifferent to life, what will happen to the living?

Anne: Neglect.

Garreth: Looking from a bird's view, everything that everybody is doing is the best he or she can do at that current moment. Would you agree with such a statement?

Anne: Yeah...

Garreth: And life that is neglected will create what?

Anne: Nothing.

Garreth: Exactly, nothing. So, if everybody is
             trying his or her best, even if that means
             failure or a big mess, how would you
             react as Fat Lady?

Anne: Nurturing. Understanding. Loving.

Garreth: Now that is some beautiful creating that
             one could do...!

             The best way to treat such dark
             emotions? Exactly like you said above,
             nurturing, understanding, and loving.

             *Use your emotions to create, try not to let
             emotions create you.*

There is much to learn from everyday situations and encounters with
people when we are open to receiving their wisdom. Often we do
not recognise this because we may be too wound up in our situations,
sorrows, pains, demands or defences. All those situations in our lives,
from the insignificant to the important, conspire to teach us exactly
what we need to be learning: patience, compassion, perseverance,
honesty, letting go, whatever is needed at the time. Perhaps this
difficult phase in your relationship with your child may be teaching
you to let go; or the homeless person you see daily on the street
corner may be challenging your belief system, showing you the
boundaries of your own generosity or compassion; or a series of lost
items may be asking you to be more present to physical reality. There
are countless books, videos, brochures, therapies, therapists, and
every esoteric, philosophical and theological nuance of 'being in the
moment'.

What does it mean to be 'in the moment'?

This is exactly what our emotions are doing, either taking us to a
specific moment, such as in a memory, or forcing us to be right here,
with the emotion, in the present. An emotion allows us to be fully
present, albeit briefly. Given this creative aspect of the human

psyche, how would you live, how would you be, how would you act and react, if every person you met, in whichever form or way, was a representation of *The Divine*? And with every single one of those meetings, those moments of confrontation, of recognising the other in every single time, you have the option to either reach out, or to withdraw. The emotions you feel actually help you to be 'in the moment', yet what you are prepared to create in every of those revelatory moments is about your essence.

∞

Understanding your essence will help you flow through life with more grace. Make an effort to look for the essence of others, especially those who irritate you or treat you badly, because it will teach you something about your own limiting beliefs about yourself, and about them. Bring healing into your own life by being present in the here and now of all encounters.

Embrace the high ideals you have for yourself. It's a crazy world out there; always attempt to discern truth from falsity and don't let the noise of the world create doubt in you! Whenever you are criticised, try not to cringe but, instead, try a *thank you* for this opportunity provided for you to grow. All obstacles and rough patches out there cease to exist or cease to be threatening, when you allow yourself to be optimised by hidden lessons as well as those in plain sight.

We all know about the perspective that, as souls, we have a bodily incarnation in this world which allows us to *experience*, right? However, perhaps the only reason why we as souls have a body *and* live on this space rock is to *carry* emotions.

Everything we do - and don't do - in life is an expression of our relationship with ourselves. This is at the basis of the concept of 'resonance'. And because we are not plain yes-no machines, but often have very complex circumstances to manage, adhere to or orient ourselves towards, it is often difficult to see behind what is presented to us in daily life, to cut through the noise and recognise the essence of it.

Allowing yourself to misinterpret encounters and then allowing a re-evaluation of it is one aspect of healing. Allowing yourself to reinforce the borders between the 'I', the 'myself', and the 'you' is another. Allowing yourself to say yes to the unknown is yet another.

It is thus unimportant how your self-expression is mirrored back to you in life. This mirror could be a person, a group of people, money, cars, cigarettes, alcohol, drugs, relationships, children, animals; more or less anything. There is no value attached to any of it, except that it is *self-referring*. If anything happens, we normally say something like 'you made me do this or that/cry/spend money/live in bad health...' However, the words you choose and the actions you take reflect on how you, and not others, interpret the situation and thus steer your own actions. Put differently, if you were to value yourself properly, the way Creation has intended it, would you not take perfect care of yourself on all levels? And if you have taken proper care of yourself at the highest level you believe is necessary or appropriate for yourself, how will you react to whatever happens outside your 'island'? Would you prefer to exert influence on the waters around you, or would you rather focus your mind, intent, and energy on fortifying the sensitive beach areas of your island?

For many people 'humility' is a very ambiguous term. It is most often associated with subordination, or even humiliation. Humility is a spiritual principle that implies a purification of the ego.

> *Humility also entails accepting yourself as you are, with your strengths and your weaknesses.*

However, many people have trouble accepting their weaknesses. They want to be perfect, the best, to achieve excellence. They don't want to admit mistakes or to show weakness. This is an aspect of our ego that makes us experience criticism or nakedness as humiliation. This negative understanding of our weaknesses is actually the opposite of humility. It is a form of ego, one that is defiant and unruly in its victimisation. Denial and defiance are control attitudes, resulting from a claim to power and perfection:

> *If I cannot be perfectly good, then I'm just totally bad.*

Why? It is offensive to the ego not to have total control. And if it cannot have this control in the context of perfection, it exercises that control in the context of denigrating and destroying oneself or others. The refusal to recognise the inner psychological reality from which one's weaknesses are being denied makes it equally impossible to see one's strengths. Lack of self-worth plays a role, but actually it is not the most fundamental cause. The most fundamental cause is the desire of the ego to control, because the ego always wants to be the 'boss'.

Truly recognising your strengths thus becomes an act of humility. Recognising your strengths means that you also have aspects that you cannot call *strengths*. Humility does not make you better or worse than you already are. Humility means recognising yourself for who you are. And you will thus stop trying to be someone else.

> *No hell is as bad as that of being trapped in your own memories, if they are bad, or traumatic.*

If you can identify with that, you need to look at how to break the cycle victimhood. Where did the cycle start? Do you have a specific memory of something that happened to you in life where you took on a limiting belief system about yourself or the world around you? And yes, this might actually be one of your most painful memories, one you have been trying to get away from for decades. However, if you find you have no way *out*, you need to try the way *in*. Go to that memory; get help pacifying that replay of a situation or event that is lodged in your mind, your emotions, or your body. As long as you are consciously or subconsciously trying to avoid the topic, the memory, or the emotion, you will be unable to be fully present: when a memory about an abortion is causing you pain and resentment, and you have a child years later, the memory will prevent you from being fully present with the child simply because guilt will poison your free flow of energy.

Cutting a lengthy psychological discussion short, look at this in terms of 'being present'. If you want to experience the dangers and the wonders of this life, you need to be present in the here and now. Stop multitasking, put the phone away, and don't be available all the time.

You need to take *repeated conscious decisions* to be present, to fill present time with all of you, and to allow present time to fill you out completely, irrespective of whether this is five minutes or five consecutive days. If you do not allow yourself to be present, you make yourself vulnerable to being treated badly, or ending up as a victim.

Modern psychology calls this *mindfulness*. Example: you have an appointment at 3 pm with your dentist, but before leaving home you think about quickly dropping something off on your way to the dentist. So you drive a bit faster, are a bit less mindful in traffic, observe less, hurry more, quickly drop off the parcel instead of perhaps chatting a bit and connecting with the other person, building another bridge; and again you are a bit less mindful. Now pressure is kicking in because you really don't want to be late. Suddenly, the only thing you are mindful about is the hurry and pressure you are feeling. You arrive at the dentist, stressed, because you engineered the circumstances in such a way that you arrived a minute before instead of five minutes before the appointment time. You squeezed yet another task into the schedule, but at what cost?

Does this sound familiar? If this is you, this is your opportunity to establish who you would be if you were to open up to possibilities. Would you be *less yourself* if you multitasked less, if you performed less, if you achieved less? Similarly, are you beset with regrets, thinking, 'If only I had spent more time with xyz'? If you are, do these regrets bog you down? 'Who would I be if I were to realise that the way I did things in my past was not ideal, or even outright wrong?' Again, be honest with yourself, state the facts, and open up to possibilities of doing things differently.

Do you feel like your life is laced with such negative cycles, that you never seem to overcome frustrations and unhappy developments? How does it feel to live life under a blanket? Are you perhaps afraid of lifting this veil and allowing the light in? How about being present, and forgetting about the loud world for a while. How about taking a conscious step to slow down and fully devote a fraction of time to something, be it an animal, a person, an opportunity, a cause?

We create defense mechanisms, views, paradigms, language, body posture, beliefs, values, and filters according to our experiences, our assessment of our current lives, the people in our lives, or the conditions and circumstances prevalent in our lives.

However, you might find yourself being stopped in your tracks when you try changing your life or circumstances. Often, this happens because your actions don't carry through enough. What you need is referred to in psychology as *bright lines* - a clearly defined rule or standard. The brighter the line, the less interpretative ambiguity and room to wiggle there is. Without bright lines, you would say something like 'Oh, I can't do it this time', and immediately this would link the present moment to a past trauma, a bad memory, some fear or other, a feeling of drowning in hopelessness, some agonising loneliness, or paralysing failure. A bright line, however, would allow you to express a response along the lines of, 'No thanks, I don't do that'. Use this to change from sacrifice to empowerment.

Remarkably, we often try to organise and run our lives with willpower. The snag is that willpower is a finite resource. A bright line will help you with that too, and most of us could definitely benefit from such in our personal and professional lives. For example, what would it *mean* to check email or social media less frequently? Similarly, what does moderate drinking entail, or what does it mean to save more, or – very popular – to eat healthy?

> *Nothing prevents you from changing your mind later. You can choose to start over at this very moment. There is no need to wait for a new week, a new month, or a new year!*

Clear statements establish bright lines ahead of time, instead of promises to yourself that are too easy to bend and discard when it comes to the actual action. Fuzzy statements make progress hard to measure, and the things we measure are the things we improve. Clear statements make actions and measures precise and obvious. Instead of having to assess situations as they arise, bright lines do the work for you, in advance. This frees up energy and willpower left over for work, relationships, and other healthy habits.

A bright line is more than just a personal boundary. Yes, at the perimeter of your Self, this could take the form of a boundary, but we establish the bright line more like 'in or out', 'hot or cold', 'fish or meat'. To those of us who don't like rigid rules and boundaries, this will be difficult. However, the aim is not to make your life more rigid, but to – at least for now – make a decision on something that you can stick to without – for now – questioning and spending energy whenever a decision-making point in life comes up.

Will this lead to you not seeing an opportunity? Yes, perhaps. Will this lead to you not living 'in the flow'? Yes, perhaps. But if you are in a position where you are pressed for mental and emotional energy, when you are feeling too tired to take decisions, then this may be the route for you, at least for now. What is important is that you find a strategy to cope with your circumstances and conditions now, and a bright line will help to cut through the turmoil, for now.

We all have our own belief systems that we derive from a variety of sources and experiences. These beliefs shape our thought patterns and emotions, which in turn influence our actions. When we act based solely on these emotions, we often behave in ways that are destructive or disengaged. If we work to expand our perspectives, we develop an ability to self-regulate, to choose to act consciously, in accordance with our higher selves, and the world around us.

How do we expand our perspectives? One of the most essential things we can do is to have *meaningful conversations*. This involves opening ourselves to listening more deeply and engaging one another whole-heartedly. Having a meaningful conversation does not mean dispensing advice or convincing another of your way of thinking; there is no winning or losing in an authentic exchange. In a meaningful conversation, we experience the value and truth of other perspectives. This gives a foundation for moving forward creatively and collectively.

Would you regard love as a universal blessing, or is this an event or a state that needs to be created in your life? Is it easily attainable? What is love to you?

If you were in a 'bad relationship with no love', or in 'no relationship and no love', or in a 'relationship with bad love', how would you proceed with your life? Would you create, or endure? Is love a finite resource, similar to willpower? Is there such a thing as 'bad' love?

∞

Peace begins with each of us. It is only after we can come from a place of groundedness, having examined our own beliefs and perspectives, that we can be present in a way that allows us to engage authentically with others. We have more in common than we can even comprehend, and *we all have the choice to respond to conflict in ways that heal rather than destroy.* Once we make that shift in our consciousness, with a sense of purpose, of how we each contribute to the bigger whole, we can finally begin to collectively bring peace to any situation and circumstance we choose!

We often find rituals to be a bad thing. Some of them are okay, you know; prayer rituals can be a nice thing and bring a family together on a religious holiday. But the idea of doing many rituals over the course of the day strikes us as archaic. It is something that 'traditional' people used to do. And thus we tend to think it's good for us that we don't have to do it because if we're going to be sincere, and true, and authentic to ourselves, we don't want rituals that tell us what to do. Then again, we seem to be creatures patterned by repetition or trauma, and some of these patterns are perceived to potentially be very dangerous. So how do we break them?

That's why you do rituals. Saying 'Bless you!' when somebody sneezes is a ritual that was established to protect the soul of the sneezing person, since it was believed that the soul momentarily left the body when one sneezed. We may laugh about such superstitions today, but we still use the ritual that was patterned in our societies and communities over 500 years ago. Often, we cloak these rituals in the guise of etiquette. Some people will cover their mirrors during a thunderstorm, or refuse to walk beneath a ladder, sit on chair number thirteen, or leave their hats on when they enter a church.

Similarly, you might be patterned by your standard responses: of fear to loud people; of isolation to antagonistic family members; of shame to condescending colleagues; or of guilt to your family member telling you about all the war time traumas and how bad the world is.

Typically, our anxieties, fears and angers are patterns embedded in our language and how we interact with others. Rituals force you, for a brief moment, to become a different person and interact with those around you in a different way. So for that brief moment, suddenly you're no longer repeating the same old patterns, you're doing something else and it is this break from habit that really matters.

For example, we may see someone and we say 'Oh hey, how's it going?' And the other person responds, 'Oh pretty good. How are you?' And we say 'Oh yeah, I'm pretty good too' and then we walk off. Now you might think, well, it's sort of silly that we do that because that's inauthentic. I'm actually not feeling pretty good right now. But if you think of this type of interaction as a ritual, it's actually a very good thing to do. And what if we did it more *fully*? You would be breaking out of the standard set of patterned responses to life and the ways we go about the day. For that brief moment, you are using language to enter a ritual space. Think structural coupling. You are connecting with someone. Things are going well. You're connecting with this person perfectly. You have broken a pattern. Done consistently, these little seemingly meaningless rituals over the course of a day or month or year break you out of these little patterns and open up other possibilities. This is why rituals matter. They break us out of patterns. We act as if we are a different person with a different set of emotions, interacting with those around us in a different way and, over time, you break these patterns.

Yes, you can rightfully argue that this 'pretending' ritual is definitely not the right ritual pattern either. However, it's the *break* that is important. Now let's go back to the greeting example. I see someone. I connect for that brief moment. Then of course that person passes and I leave the ritual space and return to my usual patterns. The point is: you keep repeating the ritual. In other words, you keep doing these little rituals over and over again. The way you greet someone. The way you shift your language if you're talking to someone. And it's those little breaks, those little shifts that make a difference over the course of time. Eventually, you begin to get a sense of the ways that those little things you do affect others. That these patterns we're playing out are bringing out predictable responses in those around us, and you begin to gain the power to alter those responses.

Imagine having an argument with someone. That person says something. It makes you angry. Your anger makes the other person angry and the situation becomes a loop of anger triggers and responses. We know this all too well. If you take these ideas seriously, all you need to do is introduce a slight shift in your standard response pattern. And even if there's not a set ritual that gives you the ability to do so, you gain something from the interaction by simply doing something different.

For example, you hold your body slightly differently, or use a slightly different tone of voice. You say something you would not normally say in the same situation. You'll immediately notice a slight shift in the other person too. You keep consciously breaking your normal response pattern. Over time – and it does take a while – you'll see that this same standard pattern that you unconsciously fall into with those around you begins to shift. And that's why this breaking of patterns is important.

Rituals create the breaks we need to enact conscious change. Over time, this shifts how you interact in and with the world and you gain the ability to work with these rituals, or work with these patterns in such a way that you longer simply repeat them. You're able to shift them and alter them according to the circumstances.

That's how, over time, you learn how to build better interactions and build better relationships. That's how to create very different worlds because you're acting in such different ways that you bring out very different responses from those around you.

This is resonance in full swing, being in the moment, and creating.

∞

There are times in our lives that lend themselves to starting something new. The beginning of a new year, finishing school, leaving a job, or changing homes: these all are times that turn our minds to fresh starts. They bring with them the energy of that event, creating a tide of change around them that we can ride to our next shoreline. But we can choose to start anew anytime. At any moment we can decide that a bad day or a relationship that's gotten off on the wrong foot can be restarted. It is a mental shift that allows us to clean the slate and approach things with fresh eyes, and we can make that choice at any time.

Starting anew is most powerful when we focus our attention on what we are *choosing to create*. Giving all of our attention to the unwanted aspects of our lives allows what we resist to persist. We need to remember to leave enough room in the process of new beginnings to be kind to ourselves, because it takes time to become accustomed to something new, no matter how much we like it. There is no need to beat ourselves up if we don't reach our new goals instantly. Instead, we acknowledge the forward motion and choose to reset and start again, knowing that with each choice we learn, grow, and move forward.

Making the choice to start anew has its own energy – it's a promise made to yourself. The forward momentum creates a sort of vacuum behind it, pulling toward you all you need to help you continue moving in your chosen direction. Once the journey has begun, it may take unexpected turns, but it never really ends. Like cycles in nature, there are periods of obvious growth and periods of dormancy that signal a time of waiting for the right moment to burst forth. Each time we choose to start anew, we dedicate ourselves to becoming the best we are able to be.

It is fascinating to see how we are all programmed from patterns that our parents inherited or adopted, even prior to our own conception, and how these play out in our own lives to make us experience and respond to the internal and external worlds in specific ways. The question is how to overcome those past, destructive, belief systems so that you can move forward in relationships, career or finances. The point is to recognise the reasons why we have these negative beliefs about ourselves. The aim is to actually start to change one's brain patterns and start attracting the things we want in life.

The thoughts, words, and actions we use to express ourselves are like the bars of our cages. They define the inside, but they also define the outside of our cages. How can we change this? We play. We engage in make-believe, pretty much like children. To the mind it does not matter whether a real or imaginary lion is standing in front of us. We enter the ritualistic space and play; all is well, slowly softening the real or perceived bars until it is safe for us to take the leap of faith out of our cage. Zoo animals seem to gaze past the bars into the distance. Animals that have been caged for a long time will seem hesitant to leave the cage if you open the door. Similarly, when people are sick for example, they are constantly reminded of their disposition, and it will leave its traces in the way they think, act, and see the world, resulting in a patterning of their behaviour or thinking, similar to a long-caged zoo animal. As soon as the brain discovers the pattern, it will remodel itself accordingly.

This is why ritual spaces are important; they break us out of this patterned space, to unlearn, to re-pattern. There are plenty of other effective tools to help us do this, but for those who don't possess the toolkit, ritualistic behaviour modification is important. For one person, this might be going to church regularly, while for another, it could be engaging with nature regularly, or for example helping with social welfare or healthcare projects, youth projects, old age support, or politics. Many would describe these as simple coping mechanisms, but when your standard response is crying, and you decide to go out and do something – yes, initially as a coping mechanism – you slowly change your standard response from being helpless to being resourceful, to being more mindful, to being more gentle or reassuring.

> By whichever means, by doing things differently, the thought patterns will follow.

Of course one could lament the painful state one is in, and then one might respond by giving a detailed account of how we got here, or one could respond with something like:

> I am exactly where and how I want to be in life.

The difference in emotional quality is immediately apparent. Watch the reaction of others. Also, observe what it does to you. What is in it for you apart from the bewildered expression on the face of the other person? For one thing, you take responsibility. You are being authentic with your response.

Firstly, *you* are the engineer of your own life. Acknowledge that with all its consequences if you can. Secondly, you are *where* you are. It is futile to pretend otherwise. Again, acknowledge that with all its consequences if you can. Thirdly, you are consciously entering a ritualistic space where you effect change within yourself and within the other.

Granted, in life we sometimes find ourselves feeling stuck, unfulfilled or dissatisfied. We feel like we are constantly hitting dead ends or passing through crossroads and paths that seem to lead nowhere. Regardless of what stage you are at in life, if you're unhappy with it, or not sure as to how to proceed, then it's time to re-evaluate. The key is to know what has the potential to make you happy now. If your current position is not what you thought it would be, then you need to move on. If you're not sure what to do next, ask yourself these 7 questions:

1. What is my favourite flavour of self-denial? Everything in life sucks, sometimes! So what kind of activity, job, career, etc. am I willing to do and put up with when times are not too promising?
2. Am I settling? We all sometimes settle for the next best thing instead of the best thing, and that makes us feel unfulfilled, like a can of soda that has been open for two days; it's there, but has no fizz!
3. What makes me forget to eat, sleep or shower? We've all had the experience where we get so involved in doing something that minutes turn into hours and hours turned into days or weeks. Sit down, and take a trip down memory lane and remember something that you used to do that completely got you in a state of flow. Look for activities that have a purpose behind them, that enthral you and keep you up for a good reason.
4. What skills, or talents am I underutilising? We all have skills or talents that we don't pay any

attention to. So, what talent or skill do you have that you can use to change your life?

5. What have I been avoiding out of fear? We all have certain things that stop us in our tracks. It doesn't matter what kind of fear it is, just do some self-analysis and aim to find if there is an area in your life where you may have allowed fear to gain the upper hand.

6. If I was told that I will die one year from today, what would I do and what legacy do I want to leave behind? We live each day with so much going on that we hardly think much about death. Not to mention that the subject just freaks many of us out. But if you're feeling stuck, then surprisingly, thinking about our own death has many practical advantages. One of them is that it forces us to focus on what is actually important in our lives and what is just busy work. So think about your legacy. How do you want to be remembered? What are the stories you want people to tell about you when you're gone?

7. How am I going to save the world? If you have watched the news lately, I am sure that you are aware of the many threats and dangers facing the world. If you're feeling unhappy and stuck, examine your values and beliefs and see how you can use them to contribute to changing the world in your own unique way. Pick a problem you care about and start solving it. Obviously, you're not going to fix the world's problems all by yourself. But you can at least contribute and make a difference and that is what matters! If you saved or helped only one person on your journey, then you might as well have saved the world, because your simple act of kindness has a ripple effect and, you never know what your actions might have done for the person you helped...

We have to realise that times of stress are also *timed and timely* signals of growth. If we use adversity properly, we can grow through it. Don't let stress diminish you. Accept the challenge, go with the flow, get all the help you need, and allow growth to happen not *to* you, but *for* you:

> *When attempting to 'clear your space', try various prayer or mantra approaches and see what works best for you. You might also want to touch your body (pat your arms, legs, abdomen, neck, head, etc.) for grounding, or widen the energy space around your body to make space for bright lines, through a prayer, affirmation, or mantra. Also, make a mental note of your mood, your fears, your anxieties and thoughts. The aim is to activate energy flow while praying (and a prayer is always positive!). When you have done this, check your mood, fears, anxieties, and thoughts again. How do you feel? Have you noticed any shift? See how this is working for you, and share it with others if you have others to share it with!*

∞

We live in crazy times; there is drama all around us. It is present in our negative relationships, pessimistic thoughts, and limiting beliefs. Drama doesn't necessarily mean 'he-said-she-said.' Drama is actually the story that you tell yourself every day, and that sometimes keeps you from thriving. So, how can you escape the drama within? How can you tap into your own abilities to *create freedom* from within, to eliminate all of the grey areas in your life, and to experience the true beauty that has been there all along?

One important issue is that of attachment. What is important to you? And what are you attached to? What does that attachment say about you, about who you are, your needs, your fears, your freedom? How many degrees of freedom do you have when you say, 'I cannot be without that person', or, 'I need this or that substance in my life'?

Can one use willpower to change this? Positive thinking? Surely that *must* help, right?

The short answer is no. The longer answer lies in the problem with positive thinking; it is just one side of the coin, and the other side is still repressed. So how about creating an intention to free yourself from drama? Have a look around you: is it *your* drama, or is it other people playing out *their* drama in your proximity? What is the drama you've experienced or witnessed saying *about you*? What if all this is a reflection of you? What do you need to realise about yourself? Why is this resonating with you? And then, the all-important question: why do you allow this to happen?

> *And if you then realise, oh wow, I am sucker for xyz, and you ask yourself 'why is that?' You try to ask yourself at least three or more times in a row 'why'. Most of the time you will end up at an intuitive answer; something which refers to 'not good enough', 'not strong enough', 'not loved enough' – although it could also be something like 'I deserve this'. The possibilities are almost endless.*

The only person who can heal this trauma is you. One way to embark on this journey is by forgiving yourself. Forgive yourself for harbouring certain memories or emotions, for actively or passively living out this or that drama, this or that substance abuse, this or that negative situation, for enduring this or that pain, and try to find out where and when you learnt to do all this. Often the source of trauma lies in the life circumstances of an earlier version of your Self. Your earlier experiences, interpretations, and self-references play a huge part in establishing the painful, limiting, or supportive belief system you carry.

> *Why is that earlier Self still active? Good question, find out why!*

How do you feel about yourself when you have any (or all) of these emotions of fear, anger, resentment, depression, and disconnect, that lead to drama in your life? What are you saying to yourself in the process?

The *thoughts* that we think create the *perspective* from which we look at things. This influences the *filters* through which we interpret the world around us. This in turn determines our *experiences*, which help to form our *beliefs* about the world. Our beliefs are what our thoughts are based upon, and so the cycle continues.

110

Obviously, if we think positive thoughts, and create a cycle of them, then we will be happier than if we were plagued by negative thoughts. However, it's not quite that simple for most of us. The result can be anxiety, a sense of being overwhelmed, and chronic ill-health. So how do you move from *empty* to *overflowing?*

Perhaps you could start with the oxygen mask analogy on an airplane; first you put on the oxygen mask for yourself, then you help others. *Talk to yourself like you would to someone you love.* But why is this important? *Your self-talk determines your self-worth.* Talking down to yourself all the time will make you feel down, worthless, useless, broken, afraid, and fearful.

Even if you cannot be *positive*, be *aware*, and use that awareness to help you *rediscover* the positive!

Despite the tribulations of the past four hundred years, we are still attached to the mind-body dichotomy of Descartes. This has led to the view that our soul 'lives' in our let's-call-it-mind, with a mechanical structure (let's call it body) attached to it, in order to successfully navigate the physical realm which we call Earth. This view has governed all mechanical-medical advances, as well as all holistic medical advances, of the past four centuries.

In quantum physics they talk of a wave function and standing wave, among many other concepts. In quantum physics, and due to the nature of everything at quantum level, observations and measurements are only statistical possibilities. Once we make a measurement, the chaos of possibilities freezes into one state, which we call measurement or observation. This is nothing more than one form of reality. Physicists call it the Heisenberg Uncertainty Principle. Once the measurement is done, the standing wave collapses again into the chaos of possibilities.

A different view could be as follows: consciousness as we know it is not a product of brain activity, but the brain is perhaps a quantum-mechanical receiver for consciousness, which originates outside the body. If we translate this to our lives – what we have in life, and what life looks and feels like – we could use the inside-out model of resonance, or we could leave all that behind and say, in clear quantum physical terms, that our reality – life – is a collapsed standing wave. As long as we attach consciousness to all of it, it simply cannot change. Remove measurement, remove consciousness, let reality return to its quantum state, and so-called change will happen, because the standing wave will collapse differently once we have a different constellation of consciousness.

> *Simple (or perhaps not so simple!) physics, but what does this mean?*

It means that dreaming up a reality will not suffice. We need to let go, stop the observation or measurement, allow change, not attach value; throw a pebble in the pond, allow the water to ripple, and only then take a new measurement or observation and notice the changes.

Too often, we only listen to the content of what somebody has to say, totally ignoring the way it is being transmitted. What about that which *is not* being said? A practical example:

> *As soon as a husband comes home from work, his wife complains about a light that needs to be repaired or replaced. Perhaps she could do it herself, but she chooses to structurally couple herself in such a way that the husband may feel obliged to do it instead. This may lead to frustrations on his side, and after a few such occurrences, this leads to an argument.*

What is happening here?

In the circles of energy medicine, most practitioners use the term 'resonance' to denote the interaction between what somebody else does and what happens within you. There is another aspect to this; whenever you refer to another person in your words, whatever you say about another person, at least in part, is a reflection of yourself. Why? Because whatever resonates with you – either negatively or positively – is important to you. Whatever is important enough to you about another person that you deem it necessary to communicate to others with words, is a statement about what their actions trigger within you.

One of the troubling aspects of resonance is the fact that *words are energy*. If you voice them, they become reality. The way you describe your world and yourself is the way you are and will be. The immediate solution to this difficulty comes from the previous chapter: forgiveness. Accept yourself, and others, the way they are. Be honest, be factual, and allow your emotions to be in the moment, then remove energy from the situation and allow healing. This is a huge responsibility, not only for you, but towards others too. Use this method in your life daily to help others!

Resonance has a lot to do with systems theory in that we need to look less at causal relationships and focus more on the system in which such activities or constellations are embedded. Instead of blaming someone, or oneself, one could try to look at the influences on that person that may have supported their action or words in the first place. In this way, 'knowing the answer' changes to 'having another perspective on the matter'. If we view our world as a huge system, with myriads of smaller subsystems, complex relationships, interdependencies and interrelationships, one question hovers over everything:

> *Is it a lower order problem, or is it a symptom of a higher order?*

Newtonian cause and effect thinking presumes a straight line between a cause and the effect it has: *if a then b*. With systems thinking, you consider the higher order system and apply *metacognition*. You take a step back to take a look at cycles and relationships. From this perspective, you spot more than one interrelated factor, each contributing in its limited way to a higher order. Countless trillions of grains of sand pile upon each other, and if you were to move through this pile, all you would see is a chaotic collection of grains. It is only when you take a step back that you see the beauty of a dune in the desert.

∞

The concept of resonance is not as New Age as it may seem; there are plenty of references to *resonance* in the Bible. Yet the idea is often treated as outlandish or outright blasphemous. If you are a Bible reader, why not reference some of these books: *James, Titus, Ephesians, Colossians, Jude, Peter, Philippians, Romans, Luke, Corinthians, John, Timothy, Acts, or Proverbs.*

In addition, the concept of *karma* is seriously misunderstood in the Western world as it is interpreted as being the punishment for past sins. On the contrary, there is no punishment. People who live in very poor conditions are not being punished for an incongruent previous life.

However, once you experience something, you have a memory of it. The experience leaves a trace somewhere in your phenomenological field (noosphere). In energy terms, the experience is in, on, or around your body, mind, or spirit. This energetic skew stays with you *until you let it go*. If you cling to this energy, it will become a lens through which you see the world or yourself, influencing your actions with the world and yourself. These actions could very well become habits or change your way of going about living your life. As long as this energy is present, and depending on whether it gets reinforced or transformed, it guides or governs your life, or informs your decisions.

> *As a human being, your job is to learn all that you can from the experience. Once the learning is complete, you need to let it all go!*

What do you expect to experience in this world, on this planet, in these times? Reality? Are we not perhaps continuously running many layers of cognitive and subconscious filters in accordance with karmic memories? Allow yourself the opportunity to open up to more possibilities. If *self-love* and *self-trust* are not in your how-to-treat-myself vocabulary, you will either experience endless frustrations or no progress at all. Trusting yourself does not mean your life will be mapped out in an instant, or that you always know what to do, where to tread, who to speak to, or how to behave at dinner with the President.

> *The aim is not so much your knowledge about the world, but gaining that all-precious knowledge about yourself!*

For a self-organising system, learning is a given. Biological memories get preserved via DNA, spiritual memories get preserved via reincarnation. What we call epigenetics is the playing out of a complex interplay and interrelatedness between these two memory systems, the environment the organism finds itself in, and the complex processes of self-perception and self-awareness within individual situations and bigger enclosing systems.

How is the choice made whether to suffer or not, and where?

The choice is not consciously made. Obviously we try to avoid painful conditions, experiences, encounters, thoughts and emotions. However, *letting go* of experiences in a spiritual sense does not mean that you are forgetting the experience, but rather that you are no longer attaching energy to it. The consequence of not letting go is a form of suffering that the Western world sees as the definition of karma. Those memories you do not let go of are transmitted into the next life on earth via reincarnation, and that constitutes karma. The presence of karmic 'memories' is similar to the morphic fields proposed by Rupert Sheldrake; they form an energetic skeleton for the enactment of life.

Each of us is a record of all the experiences we have ever had, including all the attachments and energetic constellations we did not let go of. Each one of us is a repository of our karmic memories, attempting to optimise ourselves over various reincarnations: all that, just to be here today.

Celebrate this, even if – and especially when – your life is everything but light and fluffy!

Where people in the Western world go about optimising themselves, optimising their environments, optimising methods and knowledge, people in the Eastern world are much more inclined to endure life circumstances. Western medicine uses Newtonian *if a then b* to link, for example, a lack of folic acid to neural tube birth defects. For people who do not have such scientific knowledge, the occurrence of such a birth defect would constitute a karmic burden. This does not mean that the paradigm of reincarnation and karma is wrong, but it does mean that attained knowledge is not being implemented. Does this mean that once we apply knowledge, the karmic burden disappears? Ideally, increased knowledge about myself will lead to more self-awareness, more insights, and less attachment to certain outcomes in the space we call the outside world. Mastering such non-attachment to specific outcomes leads to a state of what is colloquially known as 'flow'.

In the following chat over some tea, Andrea is discussing her unhappy marriage and how she is experiencing the push-and-pull factors of the current constellation. To experience the state of 'flow' one has to somewhat detach from wanting a certain outcome to a situation, and rather allow the dynamics to effect sweeping change. Often, we desperately want change, but cling to safe ground.

Andrea:	I believe the infidelity of my husband has affected me more than I thought it would. My life feels out of place, foreign. Yes sure, some good came of it as well…
Freya:	Yes, a lot has changed.
Andrea:	I want to feel loved, protected – I just don't know whether I want it to happen with him anymore. How did I come to feel so unsure?
Freya:	Sounds like growth…
Andrea:	I am dealing with a big struggle here, an internal struggle of sorts.
Freya:	Sure, but does the struggle stem from your husband?
Andrea:	No, not at all, it's me!
Freya:	You are struggling with yourself?
Andrea:	I am starting to realise how I can be treated and appreciated differently, better, more…

Freya: For sure! Your value system is changing, your belief system about yourself is changing; these are after-effects of your healing journey.

Andrea: But I also feel bad about it, because it looks as if I am an ungrateful cow, looking for a fight.

Freya: When patterns disappear, suddenly the world looks different, and the reasons why you did X in the past no longer apply; so X becomes unpleasant or unacceptable.

Andrea: Yes, that is happening to me right now under my own eyes. I am afraid my husband will not understand this process of mine. My vision board on how do I want to feel in my marriage with my husband: safe and secure, accepted, a solid relationship base, loved, appreciated, supported, calm, desired, understood because we communicate well, respected, laughing and happy, open communication...

Freya: OK, so change is happening. Question is, away from your husband, or possibly closer to him...

Andrea: Why am I not seeing my vision board work?

Freya: Did you have all of those wants before?

Andrea: Nope, not all of them.

Freya: So what did you have before now?

Andrea: If I look at it now, I don't feel any of that which I felt before the vision board. I am worried I destroyed it with a vision board.

Freya: The vision board doesn't destroy anything on its own; it just uncovers what is true, true for you. However, you might be a bit sensitive at the moment. Perhaps a more playful approach could help both of you to work together again?

Andrea: How?

Freya: I believe you should consider being more *in the flow*.

Andrea: Yes, I am definitely not in the flow with him.

Freya: I feel resistance from your side, as if you are trying to hold on to something, trying to salvage something. Are you perhaps trying to hold yourself back because you are afraid that if you engage in flow, you will flow away from your husband?

Andrea: Yes, I am.

Sometimes we embark on a journey in life and we are not sure of how it will turn out. Smaller journeys we might call 'projects', larger journeys we might call 'midlife', 'following one's heart', 'changing course', or even 'uprooting and replanting an old tree'. In both energy medicine and religious approaches, *truth is an essential part of success*. If you don't know whether something is true or not, drag it into the proverbial light of the Divine, and see what happens. If it perishes, it wasn't true. Sure, this can feel harsh at times, but it will be to your own benefit! You are actually employing various approaches at the same time: you establish a bright line, you empower yourself by opening up to possibilities, you orientate yourself towards truth, and you allow your Higher Self to guide you into making better decisions, informed by information that you previously used to filter out.

Whenever you are ready to do so, you should get all the help you need. This help often comes from a totally unexpected area of your life. Why? Because you are changing your energies, and you start resonating differently. You can compare this to tuning a radio to a different radio station; as you leave one radio channel, you may hear a lot of noise and irritation, but if you focus on where you want to go, you will find another channel. Ideally, you will end up being true to yourself; and if that is all you achieve, at least your life will be governed more by trust in yourself, and less by fear.

This is even more important if you have never had the opportunity to learn and trust yourself. If this sounds like you, you will agree that the absence of trust is not the presence of mistrust. It is more like an empty canvas which allows others to project their fears, ideas, hopes, plans and thinking into your life, your person, your presence. And you will always feel that these are not yours; but you lack the strength to cut them out, like bruises from a fruit.

Being kind to oneself can be interpreted on more than one level. For instance, if you have a history of beating yourself up, abusive environments, neglect, harsh words, being kind to yourself means you care for your own well-being, you create your own safe space. Where this is not the case, being brutally honest with yourself is a matter of taking stock with open eyes, acknowledging deficits, acknowledging areas where one could improve, work on, rectify, change course, fix, or simply *heal*.

∞

In psychology, there is the term 'catharsis'. In religious terminology, this would perhaps be similar to 'repentance'. However, in the bigger picture, even though this can feel abrasive and could potentially turn into self-harm – is a way of being kind to yourself, because of its cleansing, acknowledging, self-healing effect. This can lead you to think, *'Even though I am xyz, maybe I can find the strength to open up to possibility abc...'* and it also allows you to think, 'Even though I am whatever I am, I can accept myself and my emotion at least a little bit more than before'.

Whenever you would normally answer 'I don't know...' (for example, 'I don't know whether I can do xyz', 'I don't know whether I should proceed with this or that project', 'I don't know how I feel about xyz'), try saying, 'No, I don't want this...', and see how it feels.

119

Why all this saying no? Don't we already have enough negativity in our lives? Well, sometimes it is easier to first learn to say No! Learn to establish bright lines. Only when you feel more secure, will you be able to safely say Yes!

The roads we travel may be different, but the milestones we need to pass are similar. The aim is to convert stagnation into movement, to be less *affected* by change and *effect* more change, to understand why each of us faces our unique set of issues, pains, rocks, mountains, constraints, and suffering.

When confronted with an issue or problem or situation for a long time, we sometimes grow kind of accustomed to it, and we resign ourselves to the circumstances or situation. *'Who would I be if things were different?'*. Your new life always, and only, starts with that one single step. Once taken, that one single step cannot be undone, not because of higher forces at work, but simply because once you recognise a pattern, a sign, a picture, your brain will recognise it in future. For some, this one step which cannot be undone is just too much to handle; they would rather stay put and continue in their suffering. Why? Because it may feel overwhelmingly unsafe to venture away from the known. It may also feel overwhelmingly unsafe to be happy, to feel less pain, to leave behind one's internal representation of the outside world, pain and suffering included. Again, ask yourself,

'Who would I be if I did not have to suffer like this anymore?'

Others will be more pragmatic and go into attack mode:

'Even though I have been facing xyz for so long, I am ready to change now, and open up to that possibility'.

However, Nature seldom works in straight lines, except for growing crystals, so why would we expect straight-lined solutions unless they are engineered by willpower? Instead, everything develops in waves and circles (you know the expression; 'what goes around comes around'). It takes compassion for yourself as a human being, as an open, evolving and developing system, to believe in yourself, even if you think you have a lot to blame yourself for. For those of us who have gone through processes of divorce, separation, breakups, or family estrangements, at some stage the emotion of blame, guilt, or even shame rears its head – 'even though I have a lot to blame myself for, perhaps I could at some stage forgive myself (and others)'. Remember: blame really is just one of *many* competing perspectives.

For those of you who would like to approach this as a religious believer, lay all these issues at the altar, turn around, and walk away, and allow the changes to happen without your continued intervention or doing.

> *This is the promise the Divine gave to you! True forgiveness is extremely powerful.*

But what if it is not safe to take inventory of your biggest life lessons? Who would you be if you were to take inventory? The most evident path in life may actually be a lesson you need to learn and overcome.

If you would like to approach this from an energy point of view, think about energy and resonance. Even here, forgiveness plays a crucial part because it changes your energy and resonance. Find the radio station that really makes you want to dance and sing. Find out who and what you are, and who and what you are not. Learn to be true to yourself and say no to people and things that do not correspond to your inner being. Listen to inner truths and your outside world may crumble. If that happens, you may be devastated, or you take pride in –it, because it means you are taking a conscious decision to separate personal truth from falsehood, good-for-me from bad-for me, and you are learning to be true to yourself. And you can reread this as many times as you like, you will not find the word 'easy' anywhere!

> *In the past, you might also have been busy looking at yourself and your life, at others and their lives, and situations and conditions, good news and bad news, dreams and aspirations, goals and motivations with the precision of a knife, separating the conducive and the opportune from the bad and*

uncomfortable, albeit under the heading of taking responsibility, taking charge of your own life, allowing yourself to express cognitively or intuitively what is good for your and whatever needs to fall away.

You may have repeatedly heard and read about dividing: *cut this out of your life, operate there, redesign this, or do away with that*; the possibilities to do so are almost endless. The mechanism, however, is always the same: to differentiate, to take apart, or to analyse. Whether this happens by careful deliberation, philosophy, discussions, a plethora of self-help or facilitated approaches, or just 'feeling' or 'knowing', it all involves separating the *what is good for me* from the *what I don't want*, to saying *no*, separating oneself from a mix of conditions, influences, or even people.

However, as with everything in the world, there are two sides to this coin. It is also necessary to build bridges; and to walk over them. You never know when another life lesson will come your way; they seem to be layered like never-ending onion skins. Hence, you may be tasked to find love in the most impossible of places. Or you may be tasked to overcome your inner demons and reach out for support, help, freedom, health, art, ideas, stimulation: the world. For example, you could ask yourself, is my neighbour really such a dork, or am I supposed to learn something? Or, is my partner really *xyz*, or am I just looking at past appearances and not seeing his/her essence?

Life is full of appearances, but equally full of essences. Where you may have learnt to be alert to the acuteness of your inner voice, instincts, intuition, introspection and insight for being more true to yourself, you should not forget to equally open up to the world outside. Reach out, connect, build, and expose yourself to new ideas, people, and situations. Learn from others, share your experiences, and celebrate life in all its forms, figures, shapes, colours, sounds, smells, and tastes. After all, it is far too precious not to!

We all kind of live on phenomenological islands. If you share an apple with another person, each has half an apple; but if you share an idea with another person, the idea doubles. You need to build bridges so that ideas, deeds, people (and apples) can walk across them. A group of islands do not make a web of life; you need to cross the divide, reach out, help, and let the energy flow. Incidentally, this is what almost all religions teach! If you are bogged down in assuming that the position and experience of other islands is unknowable, try and allow yourself to let go of those assumptions that inform our belief system and behaviour. *Forgiveness* introduces peace into your life, irrespective of whether you want to see this in a religious sense or in plain psychological terms.

Energy needs to flow like water, and all healing modalities actually practise this explicitly. Trying to shape the flow consciously will introduce your own energy, and it will either drain you, or distort the outcome. Even here, forgiveness allows a free flow, allows truly letting go of energies, allows energy to find its destination, as in Reiki, and allows persistent healing. And then there is the mirror effect of forgiveness; it not only means forgiving somebody or something outside of you, but also forgiving yourself – for harbouring the grudge, the memory, the pain, for so many years.

So, once you give up all hope for a better past, you literally stop forcing energy onto the matter, you stop telling your body to keep on living in the trauma, you allow yourself to change, you allow the world around you to change. It might feel like surrendering, but it really is a matter of 'snapping out of it' and aligning and reintegrating your inner representation of the world with the outside, of including and integrating more of your *Self.*

Forgiveness is an experience, not a phrase you can utter like an affirmation. Every time you interact with others, you have the choice to listen, acknowledge, and let go of their words, or you can take what they are saying personally. Taking things personally is often the result of perceiving a person's actions or words as an affront or slight. In order to take something personally, you must read negative intent in an individual's words or actions. However, what people do and say has no bearing upon you and is usually based on their experiences, emotions, and perceptions. If you attempt to take what they do or say personally, you may end up feeling hurt without reason.

If you want to change something in your life, focus on the inner, and the outer will follow. So then, what does it *really* mean to overcome self-sabotage?

> *How about writing a short letter to people in your past to acknowledge and say thank you to them for bringing you to this point in your life, where you are able to reflect the way you do now. See where this gets you in dealing with a situation, with yourself, or with life! This is a process of forgiveness, and it allows you, as well as any other person involved, to heal. Genuine forgiveness is probably one, if not the most, powerful peace process we humans could possibly hope for, and truly a very precious gift!*

∞

Whenever you are ready to change something on your island, in your life, focus on the inner, and the outer will follow. Understand that, although the island is shaped by the energies that surround you, it also is shaped by the energies within you. There is a reason why you like a certain perfume, why you like certain food, why you have preferences and dislikes, why you like certain colours more than others, or why your island looks and feels the way it does. You should always attempt to be the sovereign of your of dominion. For that to happen, you need to be truthful, so take inventory of your biggest life lessons. This will allow you to break through toxic emotions that prevent you from visiting or even looking at certain areas of your island. Sure, you might ask 'Why is it important to visit a dark grotto on my island if I already know that I am afraid of it?'

The answer could be that you need to discover *all* your needs. It doesn't mean you can or should or would act on them, or live them out, but at least you are aware of them. Increased awareness will lead you to break the trance of denial, and it might lead you to discover a past hurt. The hurt in turn led you to smoking, and twenty years later, you are struggling to quit. Without addressing the hurt that led you to start smoking, you will not be able to quit smoking for good, because you are driven by one or more subconscious patterns that maintain the need to smoke.

You need to learn to feel safe in the face of fear. Technically, your stress centre gets triggered, and its only purpose is to get you, an organism embedded in a hostile world, to safety. Reframing the world into 'not so hostile as I had thought' will allow you to react differently to the same stimulus. Often, our excuses about why things are the way they are actually what keep us stuck. Once you are able to break through those layers, you are free to take power right away. When you stop fighting imagined lions, and you surrender by making peace with your pains, your life will take a definite turn towards more empowerment, more sovereignty, more strength, and more authenticity.

∞

NOOMON IX

∞

A WAY FORWARD

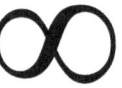

T he fact that we do not perceive our environment in the same manner as others do is an indication that truth is *relative* to the position of the individual, and thus the individual has to constitute his or her truth without losing the perspective that there is another truth which actually could counteract one's own truth. The effect of this is that truth is often moulded to fit what is most pragmatic for an individual. Truths that counteract our own worldviews are easily dismissed because it would be less pragmatic to redesign one's entire life rather than just a certain aspect. When the heliocentric universe dawned on humankind, it was extremely contentious and created a serious backlash because it counteracted the then ruling worldview.

Hence we not only constitute our own subjective reality, but we also constitute our own truth. When it comes to our truth, various ways have been devised to accomplish the same task, namely to accommodate the diversity of existence in a framework which we can supervise and which serves the need to know the world, and eventually, to justify our knowledge about the world, our activity, and our existence per se.

> *The context itself is already part of the recursive determinism which it promulgates.*

If our consciousness is nothing more than a conglomerate of very complex material patterns, then we create our own subjective world as much as the world creates its own objects, because the underlying processes are a generative force for material patterns. In effect, this notion does away with the traditional struggle for a distinction between an objective and a subjective world, as these two dimensions are incorporated into one and the same system. Our position *relative* to the entire system determines what we see.

It is thus quite unimportant to know the constituent parts of the system, or even its content. Rather, the only importance lies in intersystemic relationships. There is nothing in this world which is not part of one, or any other, system. The systemic relationships are the glue which holds together the entire world. The intermeshing of all aspects of human life really is done on several levels of interaction, even though we tend to focus less on, or even lose sight of, the bigger context.

The focus on systemic relationships makes such a theory *nonlinear* and *circular*. The dimensions of its epistemology can become increasingly obscured. Systems theory maintains that the world we live in, our system, will determine the way we see the world. Reality is not only a constant stream of potential experiences, but it is also simultaneous. It is our mind that strings these experiences into a more or less ordered and structured experience of time.

The relationship between systems is dynamic because all living systems are open systems that depend on active interchange of information. By definition, the open system needs input from the environment to establish internal differentiation and specialisation. It is only through this process that any system can exist over time. As systems are built up by subsystems and sub-elements, change in any part of a system will affect the entire system. This effect will spiral up the hierarchical order ad infinitum. This means, the more root-levelled the change is, the more profound the change in all other systems will be, and vice versa, the higher up in the hierarchy the change is, the less pressing the change will be for lower-levelled systems.

Every system has a structure, and it is the structure that implies the system's boundaries which in turn separate the system from its environment or higher-order system. The observation that not every system can be of equal status is an indication that information processing actually means *information-transformation*. There is no meaning without context - meaning cannot possibly be separated from its context. In relation to nature, there is a 'competition' of meaning within the system, and it is this competition that accounts for increased disorder. Feedback loops are an integral part of the system's functioning and are a mechanism for conveying positive or negative meaning in the context of the system's relation to its environment.

What does this mean?

130

In every respect, systems theory has the potential to be an umbrella epistemology that marks the era of *New Thinking*. There is no single 'scientific method'. While one could define the scientific method as a set of practices which scientists use to answer questions within their specific field of research or investigation, the methods employed can vary significantly. Some of the methods used for scientific enquiry are of a logical nature, while other methods are empirical in that they refer to making observations, the designing of instruments, or the designing of controlled experiments.

Complexity seems to be the keyword here, yet is not the same as *complicated*. An analysis of complex systems is concerned with the interactivity of many systems, and their abilities to adapt and co-evolve over a certain period of time. The extent to which systems inter-depend and evolve is an indication of their dynamic abilities to self-organise, and how these abilities influence the occurrences of certain events at a later stage.

We have designed highly complex systems, which transcend the capabilities of humans by countless factors, yet we find it difficult to create or allow self-attuning capabilities to such systems, in order to deal with information security and to pro-actively mitigate breaches. Instead, we use ad-hoc risk management to define information, then we define how we intend to secure such information and data, and eventually we need to use resources from other business processes such as sales to pay for the active securing of our data. And yet, despite such proliferating efforts to quantify a value chain, to identify critical success factors, or to employ methods such as the balanced score card to correctly measure and effect value within an organisation, institution or society, do many governments, organisations, and individuals around the globe end up with crippling virus outbreaks, or websites shredded by hacking. Countless billions are being lost due to industrial and other forms of espionage, lack of governance, corruption, or simply lost data.

There does not seem to be logic in this system, and yet these systems resemble how societies structure and organise themselves. Would it not be possible to align, at a much earlier point, by a paradigmatic change towards metaphysical thought that permeates cultures and societies on multiple levels?

> *The way we describe our world is an expression of the way we see our world, what we believe in, and what we count towards our culture, heritage, sciences, religion, art, identity. And yet, despite all our cultural and technological advances, people are sick, unwell, in pain, in agony, suffering across all continents, countries, and societies. We have learned to try and fix the world on the outside, whereas we really should leave causal reality and return to the synchronicity of the Divine.*

∞

Healing allows for a *reconnection* that enables the individual to grow; when you find yourself being confronted with the same problem over and over again, this is a clear indication that you are not growing. In terms of dissipative structures, the energy is not flowing; it's being stopped or held back by your body or your consciousness, leading to injury, pain, and suffering. From the previous discussion we can deduce that we are structurally determined beings, which implies that the damage or pain we incur during our lifetimes are determined not only by how we act in our environments, but also by the environments acting on us. It is of the utmost importance to not only address the physical symptom, but also to interpret the symptom within the framework of principles.

> *All the worldviews currently employed globally are totally inadequate in explaining the nature and extent of the universe, the world, our identity, our person, human nature, and the relationship we have with our environments; from the most intellectually abstracted form right down to the quantum level of action and interaction between ourselves and our immediate and distant environment.*

Just like the business world, health is not created by governments nor doctors, but by individuals. The paradigm changes require a vision of *empowering* the individual to create and maintain *individual* health and *individual* prosperity, to reduce or minimise obstacles towards goals, to embrace and actively pursue new approaches to healthcare, and to diversify, to educate, to grow. The vast global stage requires a fundamental rethinking of traditional norms and values, of traditional ways of going about doing business and living a healthy life, and our traditional ways of organising and structuring societies. It is necessary that changes occur, and changes need to be embraced and used as catalysts for accelerated growth and adaptation.

What happens if and when you run out of options on your island? What if there are so many forbidden tracks, so many dark corners, so much fear, resentment, loneliness, or despair that venturing in any direction would expose you to unspeakable terror?

We tend to keep our options open, to have a manageable range of options available for protecting us against perceived threats. Sometimes, however, life strips us of one or more of those coveted options, and our instinctive reaction is one of despair, exasperation, regret, or anger. Yet, eliminating an option may also bring us closer to our real destination. We could be annoyed about losing one of our options, or we could be thankful for not having to implement the option in our life – probably with willpower – just to find out that it wasn't the right way in the first place. It is almost as if you were using the power of a supercomputer to evaluate your plotted path, only to find that it is not worth its while.

Allowing change will often take you in an unexpected and different direction

We grow up in less rigid societies than a hundred years ago, we often abide by less rigid rules, and we are bringing a kind of chaos to previously traditional settings of uniform thinking. Diversity creates value by people being more willing and ready to change, to innovate, to question structures and processes, leading to earlier optimisation and thus possibly generating an edge over the competition. The traditional pyramid hierarchy of almost all organisations and societal structures worldwide has proven itself of only limited value. Top-down leadership is a waste of resources because it generates conflict between loyalty and other shared values, and the incessant need of organisations to innovate and redesign business processes. All these economic overgrowths and superstructures affect the lives of individuals.

You should try not to create conflict within yourself due to the absence of bright lines, or a willingness to explore your island to the fullest without endangering yourself or others.

Whether structured or unstructured, your life can become an analogy of the environment you live in. The aim is to allow the *free* flow of energy, the *free* flow of labour and market powers, the *free* flow of capital and the *freeing* (de-compartmentalisation) of previously narrow-defined social norms and conditions for you to *thrive* in, and not just *live by*. Taking care of your health can have an important influence on liberating you to rethink life and move the locus of control back into yourself. In the end, this would allow you to empower yourself to think, act, and live differently. Such freedom allows you in particular and societies at large to adapt faster, to innovate and reward citizens with sustainable economic returns. Let your island be an example to others!

Nobody is asking you to create paradise. The only person who has to live in, on, and with, the island, is you. The closer you get to yourself, the more knowledge you have about yourself, the more you maintain dialogue with your environment, stay open to change and influences, the more authority you have over the space you are inhabiting. Why would you not want that, or why would you want to pass that ownership on to somebody else?

Learn to observe, learn to listen. Often we are tasked with finding the wisdom in other people's path through life. We all have stories to tell about opportunities, dangers, despair, pain, love and hope. We all have tried and tested approaches on how to fake it, on how to make it, on how to fail, and on how to suffer. Understand that all this does not define who we are, and the day you decide to do away with a harsh cliff and create a beautiful beach paradise, there is nothing from preventing you to do so. Maintain that authority over your island, but equally understand that if you give up that authority for

134

an interpretation and enactment of your island by another person, such as a friend, a colleague, a partner, or a parent, your belief system guides your actions and emotions towards self-denial. Under such circumstances, the biggest critic of you is yourself.

> *If you need help, get help. There are many people who are more than willing and able to help you. Reach out!*

∞

NOOMON X
∞
INTEGRATING THE WORLDS

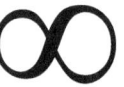

L et's take a step back and look at the human way of running one's island real estate from a higher-order perspective; let's *meta*: The aim of all meditation, mindfulness, take-your-power-back approaches, is to integrate the strengths of your left and right brain. How to go about it…?

Perhaps if we (just) choose to look at reality in a different way, one that is not governed by emotions and existing patterns made up from our core beliefs or our filters, we automatically effect change due to the mere physics of the process. A concept of *resonance*, *Law of Attraction*, or any other theoretical framework is unnecessary. Equally, it is not make-believe either, so no sitting and dreaming up a huge villa, because that is actually engaging in the *disease*. Yet it is encoding the same reality; dreaming, and not living or having, is the same kind of process.

In quantum physics, observations and the measurements of realities are only statistical possibilities. Once we take a measurement, the chaos of possibilities freezes into a specific state, which is nothing more than *one* form of reality. When we translate this to our lives and what we have, what our life looks and feels like, we can surely talk of *resonance*. However, we could also leave all that behind and say, in clear physical terms, that we need to collapse an otherwise standing wave: as long as we attach consciousness – not the same as *energy* – to all of it (meaning a specific state of the collapsed wave), it cannot change. Apparently, this is simple physics!

Imagine consciousness as a light in an otherwise dark room. Perhaps the room is endless, who knows for sure, but initially, the light is very small and you can see only a little. With experience, growth, feeling and guidance, that light becomes bigger and brighter, it can shine further and deeper into the dark room. That space the light is *en*lightening is your noosphere. Wherever the light has shone before, the unknown was made known. So then, dreaming up a reality will not suffice. We need to let go, stop the observation or measurement, and *allow* change instead of attaching value. If you compare this to the two sides of a coin, you will first need to leave your initial position of looking at the coin in order to see the other side of that coin.

Our biggest tool in the energy world is consciousness, and perhaps this is our *only* tool, our defining characteristic: consciousness. We create our own bubble of consciousness, as well as being made of consciousness ourselves. Only consciousness penetrates everything, and it keeps creating and modulating itself. We walk, talk, feel, and think, but the body really is just an extension of the brain. So if you look at such processes, constellations, conditions, causes and effects without the Law of Attraction, gratitude, or energy, you could interpret them as a matter of consciousness not attaching to a specific outcome; as long as consciousness does attach itself to the processes and their outcomes such as our five senses, the organism, the human being, remains structurally coupled to a certain energetic constellation, which we colloquially call *reality*.

Initially, the light in the dark room shines randomly in different directions. The light is aware of itself, it learns, it adds preferences to the sweeping movement, it adds fears, anxieties, anger, feelings of helplessness, hopelessness, despair, feelings of not being good enough, not being clever enough, not being strong enough; there are endless possibilities. As a result, the light intensity changes, the colour, hue, the ability to penetrate the darkness of the room, all that changes too. We call that life, living, the world around us, struggling, or failing in countless combinations of individual expressions. Layers upon uncountable layers. And yet, when we sit still and we focus on our breathing and connect to our bodies, we can enter the meditative state of just being. The world might succumb to chaos around us, the room might get darker by the minute, and yet here we are: sitting, breathing, the light switched on despite what it believes it is experiencing in the room. All that is required is for our consciousness to be as dissipative as possible:

> *Release old emotions, allow the uptake of new energy, impressions, learning, while getting rid of old stuff just as cells in your body get rid of CO_2 and nutrient wastes, making way for the next red blood cell to drop an oxygen molecule at its membrane. If this did not happen the cell would be damaged within minutes and perish.*

However, on a consciousness level, we humans tend to believe that adding that pair of shoes, this house, that car, or that substance into our light, will make the light stronger, bigger, invincible, or just better. We stuff our faces, we shop until we drop, or we consume until all is consumed. The experiences of humankind have shown that this is a pit of fallacious reasoning upon which entire industries and worlds are built. There are those industries that provide those items, but there are also those upcoming industries that nudge, persuade, and help millions of consciousness entities around the world to realise that the established ways of dealing with trauma and pain is less than ideal, if not wrong.

Everything really just *is* consciousness. Understand that everything is one; there are no differences even though our brains make it appear as if the world is a world of differences and separations. When our consciousness leaves the divine Oneness, it vibrates into a condensed form. Seen from a different perspective, we call this matter, reality, life. And yet, it is really nothing but consciousness modulating itself into a specific form. To that extent, the old Vedic insight that this world is a simulation within a simulation is quite correct, but not in the way people understand the quote, and not in the way we understand the term *simulation*. The simulation happens in each of us. We have no choice but to experience the world in an exclusive, subjective way. Sure, we listen to others, their experiences, and we try to abstract a common denominator that we might – eventually – call *objective reality*. Indeed, one of the bigger questions is: would the universe still exist if we removed all observers from it? We need to realise that life is not the way it *presents* itself to us, even though this apparent non-existent reality can also cause an organism to perish. At least on a certain level, the experience of life is mediated by consciousness.

> *Everything that is happening in, or around us, is a way of modulating our consciousness!*

In addition to quantum complexities and absurdities, much psychological and social research has shown that we need to engage our brains to the fullest. While our *left brain* is responsible for our analytical and methodical thinking, our *right brain* takes care of our creative and artistic modes of thinking. Ideally, you would want both functional aspects of your brain to channel, pass, transfer, and funnel information and energy equally and freely between them.

∞

Enough of this psychobabble! How could this help you run your island more holistically? Well, look at your life – the 'issues', the 'problems', the 'pains', and all the 'no-go areas' – and start with a left brain item or list of items. Pass it to the right brain by finding and attaching a picture that represents that item. For example, the issue of not having enough money could be translated into a picture of walking barefoot somewhere, as it is raining coins that pave the way, shining in the moonlight like an illuminated pathway. The combination of an analysed item and matching that representation with a feeling that is associated with the item will create an *intention*.

Use the intention to effect the change: suddenly, stuff happens, reality shifts. Some call it healing, but if we strip away all the modelling tools such as fancy wording, calculations, rules, and all the other stuff we come up with, and we just look at the physics, then there is no such thing as healing in the traditional sense: Your *reality* represents the constellation and relationship between you and yourself. Intent is the change you exert on your inner representation of the outside world. In Western societies, we learn to try and change the outside world to our liking, but this is a cumbersome task, requiring enormous amounts of energy, of willpower, of goodwill and positive thinking, or a combination of all of them. Unfortunately, all these powers are resources that get depleted, like your ability to concentrate, or perhaps even consciousness per se. In addition, because everything and everybody in *your* life is connected to *your* consciousness, the only domain you *really* have control over is your inner world. Be alert to how we use colloquial language to denote that inner space as *world*.

> *Your primary concern with effecting change in the world is yourself, your mode of operation, the constellation, disposition, structure, extent, colour, form, mass, composition, of your own consciousness. Self-care is being aware about yourself, your emotions, your noosphere, your unique constellation of elements of consciousness.*

Connecting to the energy wherever it sits in your noosphere, irrespective of whether you call it information field, morphic field, auric field, or any other term, is at the core of all modifications of consciousness. It doesn't matter whether you call it healing or anything including the term 'quantum'. This actually *means* that we also have at least one, probably countless, relationships with our worst emotions, our enemies, our hopes, dreams, failures, angers, feelings of helplessness, and basically *everything else*.

However, the take-home message here is that *the less you think, the more powerful the outcome*. In essence, creating an intention based on your strength is more powerful in creating change than intent based on your one or many deficiencies. We probably always and universally experience deficiencies as a *lack of something* that we try to add from the outside, in all its humorous or pathological *variations on a theme*:

THE SEPARATION OF THE SOUL FROM THE DIVINE.

This is probably the primary fear upon which all human life on this planet is modelling itself.

George:	If one is afraid of getting no as an answer, can one ask the Universe to take it away? Surely that would allow one to focus on the yes instead of the no. I would need this to excel in my job, to acquire new clients, and to generally be successful.
Marc:	I would recommend you first ask yourself 'why?' five times in a row. Like in 'I am afraid of a no from person *x*'. 'Why?' 'Because of *xyz*' 'Why?' 'Because it will make me feel *abc*' 'Why?' etc. Ask 'why?' five times in a row and see where it takes you.
George:	It might get personal! It will get to 'I am not worthy'. That I know instinctively!

Marc: Sure. You will see that it is never really about the outside but about your inside.

George: Should I focus on being worthy? Worthy of success? Worthy of landing a big deal? Etc.

Marc: Oh for sure. Why are you saying you're not worthy of anything?? Who taught you that? The Divine definitely didn't.

George: Other people's choices and actions based on their own beliefs.

Marc: Exactly, even though *you* learned to see them based on yourself.

George: Yes, and that is what one always struggles with, and forgets to keep in mind! On top of that comes the inner struggle, energy blockages and stuff...

Marc: There you go!

George: Ok.... long road but it starts with a single step, right? Wouldn't it be nice to be completely free of that?

Marc: And this was your original question: If one gets the fear of a no as answer to inner questions, can one ask the Universe or the Divine to lift this from you?

Consciousness also means that we are feeling *energy* as *emotion*, and for that we need a body. Most of us experience emotions as something very tangible; they may have colour, shape, location, intensity. Our noetic dealing with this includes our conscious and subconscious action, reactions, values and beliefs – information that we gather from yet to be discovered channels, organs, organelles, fields, sources, or constellations of smaller or grander scale:

Lucy: Hi, I had a huge fight with hubby this morning. He stormed out and is on his own mission. I definitely don't want to run after him.

Julia: OK!

Lucy: He of course feels as if everything is my fault, but I feel this is a bit unreasonable.

Julia: And how are you feeling now?

Lucy: First I felt like I would have a panic attack, but then I calmed down. I will just focus on my own stuff. Is it OK if I don't run after him? Maybe he needs space and time as well? What do you think?

Julia: He can be as stressed as he wants, that doesn't mean he is right, and even less that he is always right.

Lucy: I think he has a point, to a certain extent, but there certainly are ways to handle this better. I did say I was sorry, though. Then again, it wasn't the end of the world either. Oh well....

Julia: Do you think this fight was damaging to your marriage?

Lucy: Yeah, perhaps. That's something I always worry about. Then again, which argument is not damaging? In the end, I didn't give him space to calm down :(What should I have done differently?

Julia: So, what you are saying is, you triggered him big time?

Lucy: Yep.

Julia: Level 1: Why? I am not judging, just asking. Say whatever comes to your mind first.

Lucy: I don't share his values on certain things, and I did not communicate something to him.

Julia: Level 2: Why?

Lucy: Because I thought our family was more important than somebody else's family!

Julia: Level 3: Why?

Lucy: I wanted to spend time with him instead of spending time with somebody else.

Julia: Level 4: Why?

Lucy: It felt like other people were more important than us.

Julia: Level 5: Why?

Lucy: And I was not worthy of him making a decision for us and of spending time with us. I rebelled, but at the same time made his life a bit harder. And by not being as warm as I normally am.

Julia: And that makes you feel how?

Lucy: Angry and rejected.

Julia: Why?

Lucy: He says, if he is so angry with me, he has no sex drive, and he is not warm and friendly towards me either. I am not special to him. Just nothing. Or I don't respect his values and I am selfish.

Julia: Does he respect your values?

Lucy: Not always.

Julia: And, is he selfish?

Lucy: Yes.

Julia: And how does that make you feel?

Lucy: It makes me extremely angry! If he was perfect, and I was an idiot, I would run after him for sure! But I am not, and neither is he!

Julia: So what would happen if you were to run after him?

Lucy: I would degrade myself. And become worthless.

Julia: Why?

Lucy: Because it would make me feel weak. I would have to bend. He didn't understand my concerns, or what was important to me. Battle of wills.

Julia: So perhaps he realises that you have changed, and you are not the same as a year ago. Perhaps you could come up with a list of what has changed, so you have it with you during your next calm conversation with him. He needs to understand your shift.

Lucy: OK. I simply don't understand how other people would see you as family, but your own family has this kind of dynamics. So, I am starting to understand that friends become family.

Julia: I do understand; it is a fallacy to think that our partner, or our family, always stays the same, while we allow friends to change, because – in the end – a friendship can cool off if that person changes too much for our liking. Difficult to do with family. And suddenly, things are all sticky and unpleasant.

The important thing here is the observation that what we see, hear, taste, touch, and smell are not mere reactions to an outside world, but are in fact simulations of such a world. Whether we call it a *matrix* or *simulation*, a *phenomenological island*, *brain and body dichotomy*, *individual versus the universe*, or anything else for that matter is not important, except for the requirement that we need to *break* that simulation and reconstitute it on a different footing. This is sometimes a belief system, a different perspective, a fact-check, a catharsis, or perhaps something bigger and more thorough.

Due to this constant internal simulation game, the brain is used to predicting and analysing what happens next, and if necessary, or preferred, it brings forth a unique mix of congruence and incongruence that serve as justification for later actions. Obviously, that brings a new layer of complexity and difficulty to the underlying processes. Thus we do not have what we colloquially call *issues*, but rather strategies that are or have been an answer to a unique constellation of perceived inner and outer conditions, emotions, people, constellations, pains, etc. Such strategies are thus always situational, and the aim is to let the strategies go once the situation has been outlived.

∞

Highlighting the aspects of congruence and incongruence with reference to disease and health, thriving and declining, fear and prosperity, desire and defeat, elucidates the need to create energy pathways between the internal and external world that allow flow and healing, pathways that foster the dissipation of energy uptakes by structurally coupling with the environment. Thus, the congruence model could be used to explain the success of somatic therapies without referring to *energy, holographics, morphic fields, meridians,* or any other postulate of energy. It might be much easier to understand for the normal user than referring to energy, of which every practitioner in the field has his or her own unique understanding and experience. Perhaps the model is more to explain the process than the intervention. Ideally, we would find a simple tool or process to transform our incongruences while still engaging all of our senses, and emotions, as well as left brain and right brain faculties:

> *Peter is suffering from persistent lower back pains that just won't go away, no matter what he does or how he tries to alleviate it.*

He has been to a string of practitioners to no avail. It turns out, the pain is linked to the betrayal of his former partner a few years earlier. The concept at stake is that of 'painful persistent pattern'. Meaning, this is how he confirmed his own belief about another person, something like 'This is how much I love you, or, this is how much you betrayed me, and this pain is there to remind me – and you – of the impact of your actions'.

Whether as a loved one or perpetrator, one would need to find a more positive way for him to remember the other person. At this moment in Peter's life, the lower back pain is a much more intense and yet more manageable reminder of his former partner. Why? Because, unlike the ex-partner, you can take the pain with you wherever you go. To reach the point of it becoming a happy memory, he would have to let the memory of her go, let her be, and move on. In addition, who would he be if he were to let go of the (literally) painful memory?

Humans often carry emotions on the outside (meaning *in the body*), leading to bending, bouncing, flowing, blocking and all sorts of physical and mental contortions. This can give rise to all kinds of body forms, morphologies, voice and posture patterns, or new layers of thought or emotional patterns; all to which, in turn, react with all kinds of reactive behaviour, layer upon layer; yet seen in its holistic connectedness this is such a beautiful symphony of consciousness.

We need to understand that we are running on consciousness instead of Darwinian biological functioning. Consciousness is the substrate upon which the entire universe is built. One level up, and quantum physics talks about energies that pop in and out of existence, another level up we talk about elemental particles, atoms, molecule, and so on until, further up, we can make out entire galaxies. In essence, however, we are consciousness that modulates other energies around us. We call that reality, or the physical world. We take on energies, and don't give them off again, energies such as emotions from other people, objects – that are also just energy – that we unfathomably believe we need, and myriad variations in between. In a way, our consciousness is like a magnet, and this is perhaps where the postulated Law of Attraction comes from. Consciousness is the basis of *everything*. There is a built-in bias, a gravitation of *everything* towards embodied consciousness.

When we see the world and ourselves in these terms, *thought and energy hygiene* are more important than ever before. We will start seeing our energetic pollution of an energetic space that is more profound than what we colloquially describe as energy. Saying that we are souls having a physical experience is not enough. We know how to keep the body clean, but we know almost nothing about consciousness.

Generating intention is a pure expression of consciousness. Intention is not the same as willpower, on the contrary, but basing our intention on something we *want* is the wrong way of creating. It is based on a need perhaps, a want, a desire, a deficiency, meaning:

> *You are standing in front of a closed door, you generate intention and hope to trigger a Law of Attraction-like process for a key, but guess what? It is not working. We have all tried it, countless times. Why is this not working? Because your intention comes from a position of deficiency. The real magic happens when you can generate an intention based on your strengths. Instantly, you might find that you have outgrown the lock and key problem.*

And yet there are people who will tell you that if they pray to God, He provides, and they find themselves in a life of abundance. So one thinks about that too, and we tend to postulate even more 'energy laws' such as the ubiquitous Law Of Attraction, this time basing it on the perceived abundance and, hey, 'gratitude' comes into play. But is this really the case?

Where exactly is this healing space?

There is no such thing as energy in energy medicine, but only consciousness. We all are consciousness workers, we walk and talk and do, we operate on consciousness all the time. Changing five, or fifty, five hundred, or twelve thousand eight hundred and thirteen configuration points in a total dataset of many trillions allows our consciousness to perceive differently. How many points do we need to change? Nobody knows...

We modulate consciousness with nootropics and psychotropics, with mood enhancers and antidepressants, but we equally modulate consciousness with money, bricks, gold, New Age thought, religion, stardust, unicorns, Ascended Masters: literally anything. Of all possible realities, the one we perceive is the one that matters at any given moment. And yet we aim higher, we aim to think more deeply, we aim to feel more intense. We drive ourselves to optimise beyond the physical norm of the day, we run after many different truths and attach ourselves to many different gurus. In the end, we know nothing except for that which we *know*. Life does not operate linearly, but in self-referential circles.

Understand that everything is forgivable. Understand that nothing is permanent. Understand that things never are the way they seem. Understand that the only state you need to be in is to be the *most of yourself (your Self)*. Understand that you need to free yourself energetically from everything that binds you, prevents you, prohibits you, keeps you small, weak, or merely functioning.

Remember your true nature, your essence, the creative strengths within you, and use those powers to *create* every single moment of your life as a human being. We don't learn this anywhere. Some will come to realise this after a severe illness, others will have intense 'aha' moments, and yet others will experience the blessings of Grace.

Understand that the most important question in the universe is: who am I? And not how am I? Observe your own consciousness taking you to your truths, *allowing* and *accepting* what is shown or realised. This is your first step in clearing your filters, patterns, layers, or defences. Your question about 'who am I?' is always based on your strengths, simply because:

The answer to 'who am I?' is always I am!

Is it bad not to be able to play the piano? Not at all, but neither is it bad to not consciously create your life. It is just that, an *un*created – or, to be more precise, an *in*completely created life. So, truly, while you are here, you might as well create all you can!

151

Enlightenment comes from engaging with the world around and inside of us, the dark room, with another, and for another. At the same time, nothing matters, because everything *is*. There is no level, no higher or lower, no better or worse, no good or bad. Consciousness is *the primal reality*. Everything is an ineffable symphony of consciousness creating itself in all conceivable forms, sound, light, or matter. The beauty of it all, the symmetry, the space, the diversity and yet the unity is breathtaking.

∞

Your island is equally a construct of consciousness. It is the perfect illusion of *being*. It is so perfect, that you take reality as physical reality, with physical consequences, physical laws of nature, mathematics, and everything else we 'discover' in this world.

Practise taking a step back and looking at the bigger picture, and most symptoms are just that: symptoms. Also consider whether any symptom and condition is a matter of self-worth, self-respect, self-love. Think about substance abuse, toxic relationships, cultural conditioning, or lifestyle issues. At any given moment, you will always be at the end of your path. Had your path been different, your current position would also be different. Whichever path it is, everything on that path has led you to this point in time, whenever or wherever that may be.

When we accept and make peace with that, we don't try to redo past actions, we don't attempt to make things different. Instead, we come to understand that life could always be a notch fuller, a notch more creative, a notch more representative of what is inside ourselves. It is less about created actions and situations, and the potential for pain they bring, and more about the lack that comes from having created neither happiness nor pain...

The exploration of your island space will take various paths. Many elements will come together, some paths you will follow religiously, others spiritually, while other corners you will explore in a scientific way. To argue that only one is valid is extremely limiting, simply because the *Gestalt* is more than the sum of its constituent parts. For one, you have quantifiable data and objective measures that can be repeated always and everywhere, given that all parameters which could influence the measurement process have been analysed and specified in the research design. This is the predominant research methodology of all natural sciences.

However, you also have qualitative data that is about evaluating, measuring, and understanding psychological matters, subjective opinions, goals, beliefs, and so on. Here, often, you will talk about the quality of a situation, circumstance, or emotion. For example, you will talk about a *cold* heart, a *stiff* atmosphere at a reception, or a *sad* realisation. The attempt to understand the complexities of a subjectively experienced, but socially constructed, reality requires an understanding of the context within which such processes happen and meaning is imbued in a multitude of processes and relations. Equally, you need to understand that all your inner life, all your emotional, psychological, spiritual processes are happening within a context, and part of the process of learning to navigate your noosphere is to discern foreground from background, occurrence from context, and data from noise. Despite being an island, you are not isolated, nor do you exist in isolation. When we replace our 'actor on a stage' thinking to a cyclical thinking where everything is in a relationship to other things or persons, our approach to life changes on a very fundamental level.

The ability to shift contexts and correlate one set of information with another brings about new fields of interest. Open yourself to discovering and living interconnectedness *on* and *about* your island, and how to bridge your island with those of others. Understand that the way you see your world is an expression of culture, a paradigm that informs the methods you use, the interpretations you derive, the way you integrate it all, and the way you see yourself. Every bridge you establish to another island is like a door to a new reality, to that other person's way of interpreting what he or she calls reality. It is yet another path through the maze we call life. And who knows: we might learn something new from the way others find their way!

Use your island to create all of yourself, to be in contact with all your inner facets, your feelings, your strengths and weaknesses. Be the sovereign over all your land. Bring your shadows into awareness instead of locking them up in the dungeons of your subconscious. Be the blue-collar knowledge worker of your own dominion, empowered by knowledge about a spectacular island, second to none. Acknowledge the beauty and complexity of it all, nurture it, appreciate and love it. No relationship is as important as the one you have with yourself, and if you need help to connect with suppressed material, be encouraged to do so. Help *is* available!

Have the courage to walk new paths on your island, take different paths through the jungle, and approach the cliffs and abysses from all sides. There is always a way forward. Sure, it can be painful if you are stopped in your tracks, but overcome the pain quickly and walk a different path. There is always a path to the Divine. Those who cannot appreciate your island cannot appreciate themselves. Their understanding of your maze is as limited as is their understanding of their own maze. Redirect those currents to those areas of your island where the bedrock is especially hard, and keep the pristine beaches for those visitors who don't litter or dump their own energies onto your shores. Clear your fields of weeds, especially those that visitors from other islands have dropped there. They are literally outsourcing their stuff to another space, probably because their own space is already overgrown. Create your island as you would like your life to be. Change direction when you need to.

> *Your entire life is a spiritual journey. It is not to find anything, but to exhaust you to the point of surrender, to the point of intentionally transferring control to the Divine and allowing yourself to be guided.*

∞

154

NOOMON XI
∞
NAVIGATING CHANGED LANDS

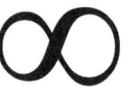

L et us return to your island, that beautiful, stunning piece of art:

It is the most unique and enjoyable symphony of varying densities of frequency, vibration, resonance, and an immaculate play of energy so intricate and bold, yet timid and adorable, that one could spend lifetimes being you.

Now, for a moment, consider walking across this island, and suddenly there is a lion right in front of you: what will you do? Yes, running, fighting, or freezing on the spot are your normal responses. Your stress centre is triggered big time. Your amygdala, as part of the brain stem, is a whopping 500 million years older than your prefrontal cortex, the brain area where you decide what to buy for your next dinner. Your stress centre is responsible for keeping you, as an organism in nature, safe.

Naturally, if you were to see the lion while it is still 500m away, your chances of survival are much higher. So what does your brain do? It will be trying to identify and analyse whether the grass is all bent in one direction or how are the colour shadings in the savannah? From which direction is the wind blowing? Is this lion territory in the first place? Did the birds stop singing? Are there any lion footprints? Are there other animals unperturbed by danger? In short, your brain is looking for patterns, and it still does so today.

Now think back to your early childhood, when you were around four years of age, possibly earlier or later. You are playing outside in the garden, with water and mud and sticks and stones and unicorns, totally absorbed in your play and totally creating worlds in your mind. Mom is in the kitchen making some food. At some stage she calls you. You have been playing for hours, are really hungry, so you drop everything and storm into the house. As you enter the house, your mum says something like: *uh uh uhhhh...* while waiving her hand frantically, indicating to you not to enter the house. Can you remember what your mum used to say? It was probably something like, 'go and wash your hands'…

So far so good. But what you might have heard is:

Unless I do what mom says, she doesn't love me.

Naturally, this is an entirely different basis for your life. You do everything the parents want you to do, you do everything the teachers at school ask you to do - you might even have been very social and popular at school.

Later in life, you have your first girlfriend or boyfriend and you resort to literally doing everything for the other person, and surely, it doesn't work out. You keep trying to do your best and make huge efforts but with little return.

At some stage, you finish school and start working, and you always have to deal with a boss who grinds you, so you switch jobs often. At some stage you are in your 30s or 40s, and you turn around, look at your life, and ask yourself:

Why do I always have 'these' kinds of men or women in my life, what am I doing to attract these or that or xyz?

So you head over to the therapy island and try to find those three, five or ten seconds mom said whatever she did back then, and you will most probably also remember them. In contrast, your memories about what you got for your birthday when you were 5, 7, 9, 11, 13 (or other) might be all gone. Why does your brain spend energy 24 hours a day, for decades, keeping those few seconds mom said *xyz* alive, while other memories your brain just drops and lets go of? What is so important about those few seconds, that you remember those even decades later?

The answer could be that behind those memories lurks an insult, an injury, a pain, or an injustice: a lion. And that lion could be something like – 'I am not good enough', 'I am not slim enough', 'I cannot do math', 'I am not allowed to sit open-legged and whistle like the boys' (if you are a skirt-wearing girl), 'I am not xyz' – there are a gazillion possibilities here....

As long as that proverbial lion is sitting there, triggering your stress centre, the brain will build a protective layer, an early warning system, around that lion. A random (but mostly not so random) trigger can come along - the taxi at the traffic light, the cashier at the supermarket, your child, your partner, your colleague, your boss, your teacher, something a random person said, a look that lasts a split-second; and that trigger will enter your brain through eyes or ears, pass through your filters, and within a fraction of a second, that pattern gets activated because the stress centre perceives a lion that is literally right in front of you!

Once those patterns are active, there is not much you can do – traditionally - to fix it. People will try to use positive thinking, they will try to 'get over it', or they will employ willpower. Yes, willpower is popular, but it does not work, it is an exhaustible resource. Every addict has the demand by society or on himself to use willpower to overcome the addiction. Similarly, food is a major painkiller for humans, so is shopping, sex, relationships, alcohol, drugs, money, or luxury items.

Clearly our current approach to addiction or overcoming tiny, small, or large trauma is simply wrong, or incomplete at best. People do not have this or that *issue*, there is no such state or thing or condition we colloquially call 'issue'. Effectively, they are coping mechanisms. The behaviour or emotion came to be because that individual had to make sense of an external constellation of how the world around looked, felt, sounded, tasted, or smelled like, and an internal constellation of a more or less major mix of emotions. Here, an obvious incongruence plays into the complexity of what we would call a *disorder*, however benign.

Safety is a condition, not an occurrence.

Does the '*unless I do what mom says, she doesn't love me*' above constitute a trauma? Very possibly so, yes. Why? Because perhaps nobody took the time to apologise for the harsh response when the child entered the house, or took time to explain to the little child that for these reasons there are those rules, and that the child is still loved very much despite the mistake or error. Small things like this easily get lost in the daily stress and routine, or simply for the reason of negligence. For some, these small insults and injuries pile up and accumulate in what is later termed *developmental trauma*. Whichever way it turns out, we are littered by such small injuries, from home, from school, from growing up, from virtually any corner of our lives.

People deal with these countless injuries differently - some people can go to war and come back as if nothing had happened, while others will suffer for the rest of their lives from it. We easily speak lightly of others, especially those that are having a hard time, stuck in addiction, or stuck in freeze state due to some or other lion, and we quickly say something like 'wow, what's wrong with that person?'; whereas we should really consider the history of that person, as in 'wow, what happened to you?'. If you were panicky afraid of spiders, no amount of talk therapy will be able to help you. In fact, you already *know* that the fear is irrational, but it is just too strong for willpower to overcome that emotion of fear. If at all, your willpower will suffice for a few seconds only. However, there is nothing wrong with your system. On the contrary, it works exactly how it is supposed to work - keep you safe. For the stress centre, a real lion and an imagined lion is the same. Somewhere in all of us sits a lion, and the defense mechanisms, the coping pattern, the resulting belief about the world or about ourselves generate a new layer of activity and emotions that give rise to new perceptions, and thus new realities.

From the vantage point of your younger Self - whenever that was in your past - these patterns make perfect sense. Maybe not today anymore, but back then, they normally represent the only possible way forward from an internal and external constellation. And surely, people may even develop a stomach pain, a cough, a headache, or even very elaborate systems of disease or disorder. As such, every disease has at least an emotional component that one can trace back to one of these patterns or belief systems. Normally, the body develops symptoms that correspond to the snapshot the body and mind took at the moment of trauma.

Nothing changes as quickly as the past.

160

Yeah right, easier said than done.

Ideally, you would want to seek a practitioner who will facilitate your growth, who provides and keeps a space for you to feel secure enough to revisit those memories in order to basically *reprogram* your physical body by releasing trauma, patterns, belief systems, and even pain from your noosphere. A lot of things happen in your body when you release old pain, wounds, insults, and injustices. For instance, your entire immune system normalises just by removing hidden lions from your noosphere, to which your nervous system reacts with a basket of different hormones.

Allowing such healing requires you to find the courage to *be in the moment*, to allow yourself to witness a multitude of factors come together to give rise to your memory. To help you with that, it is important to understand Kairos. Kairos (καιρός) is an Ancient Greek word that refers to a critical moment where opportunity directs the flow of occurrences. In contrast to chronos (χρόνος) the term Kairos has the sense of significance and of spiritual implications.

> *Kairos refers to that conjecture in life where energetic constellations come together to condense and enrich that moment in time, where you are truly present; where you allow all that comes together to express itself unfettered in an explosion of inspiration or 'things falling into place' miraculously; where you allow the realisation and experience of an unprecedented density and richness of life to reflect the beauty and symmetry of synchronicity beyond our fathomable causal reality.*

However, once you let it go, it can vibrate and be just the way it wants to. Simply because have, and have not; want, and not want; be, and not be; all encode in the same way – they are just different aspects of the space of being different sides of the same coin. Energy and information encode in the same way; health and disease also encode in the same way, just viewed from different directions. Pain is not pathology, although most healthcare is based on such a notion. The causality you are seeing or experiencing is merely a specific aspect of the reality of synchronicity. Attaching value means attaching filters, directing energy towards it, influencing the state of a vibrational constellation.

∞

7h3 gr3a7357 73chn010gy h1dd3n fr0m y0u 15 y0ur 0wn c0n5c10u5n355!

∞

Being in a world as material and fixed as ours is a mixed blessing. For one, having a corporeal life, an embodied life as consciousness is truly a blessing. Everything is here to help us, literally, even though we tend to see the projections only instead of the projector. Problems are really not problems when we allow ourselves to change, to adapt, to restructure, to regroup, to let go of stale beliefs and values, and so much more. When we engage with the world in such a way, we add a certain fluidity to our *beingness*. In a way, we remain stuck in front of a mountain until we realise there actually is none. In those moments where we grow like that, life changes, this world changes, and we start to construct that which we call *reality* a little bit differently. In contrast, in the energy world everything and anything is possible in an instant. Here, we create continuously. Most of what we create, though, is noise. Every thought, no matter how fickle, is promptly executed and has an endless string of consequences beyond the border of our earthly world.

All this is truly powered by the consciousness of the Divine.

The harmonics and symmetries of energy world are breathtakingly magnificent. There is absolutely no wrong whatsoever. Nor is there a wrong note, a discord frequency, a negative vibration, just an everlasting and unfathomable symphony of total interplay. The presence of this vibrating consciousness feeds into all matter, all existence; it builds all structures, all spaces, and all being. Everything that exists resonates with this consciousness, and yet it is embedded in it.

This is a world we have absolutely no clue about; we never learn about this, until the day we do. When you are allowed to peek through the fabric of reality, the machinery behind all of reality – not just ours – it is a deeply spiritual experience. Everything your consciousness accumulates in terms of physical matter, experiences, energies, vibrations is a cloud, a drop of ink in otherwise clear water. Over the millennia, these ink drops aggregate and give you a tainted view of Creation. We call it reality, and you may be content with the monochrome view of all that is for many lifetimes, yet there comes a point in your existence where you are prepared to *will* truth into your noosphere.

> *For this you need to let go of (limiting) belief systems, live your (inner) truths, shine your (soul) light, let go of past 'stuff' and negative experiences, acknowledge your path, wanting to be exactly where you are right now, and fill the vast space of the moment with presence.*

After you have failed so many times, and when you are ready to try creating your life in accordance with your inner truths, there is no stopping you. You will also come to realise that there is no body-mind dichotomy, there is no male-female dualism, and there is no up-down trajectory. The oneness of all perceived or postulated separations is a greatly liberating experience, but it bears important consequences for your current life:

> *What happens without your permission reveals where you are not self-aware: your Self is incongruent with that which you traditionally describe as outside of yourself.*

The aim here is not to control everything, but because *energy flows where consciousness goes*, you want to be *aware* of your noosphere; being aware of what goes on around and on your island will allow you to be present. Instead of repressing emotions, even the negative ones, you are tasked to accept them all, reintegrate them into your Self, convert traumatic memories into memories from which you can learn, memories that in the larger scheme of things actually make sense and that brought you to this point in your life - right here, and right now.

The Divine is like the *overtone* of the universe. It is that singular vibration that originated like a ripple on a quiet surface of a lake, carrying and creating all the information, form and structure for everything following thereafter. This does not necessarily equate with the Big Bang, which we are not sure was like science theorises it to have been.

When you put a singing bowl on your body, the body will absorb all lower frequencies, and what remains after a while is one or more overtones. Singing bowls are hard-coded on a specific set of frequencies, but ideally, the remaining overtone(s) will be unique, like a fingerprint for every object. This universe absorbs certain frequencies because the compaction of vibrations into what we call matter creates resistance.

As you train your third eye and brain with the overtone(s) of your body, you will be able to heal anything within your own body. As you train your third eye and brain with the overtone(s) of another person, you will be able to heal that person. As you train your third eye and brain with the overtone(s) of other realities, you will be able to look into those dimensions and realities. Your body is an extension of your brain; it is not a separate entity. Our minds are capable of seeing other realities and entities, but the body is kept in this reality by the density of the vibrations it experiences in this reality. However, if you do 'braintrainment' correctly, your entire system will believe in the validity of another reality your mind is seeing, and will thus participate accordingly. This will enable you to communicate with any entity, anywhere, in any reality, once you know the governing overtones of those realities. You can dial in to those frequencies like a radio tuning into a specific station.

When everything is vibration, frequency, and information, then clearly it does not matter whether I give you a physical tablet, or just the *information content*. Unlike in our daily so-called physical world, the *only* tool you have in the energy world is consciousness. If ancient Hindi literature talks about chakras, then those so-called energy centres are really *centres of consciousness*. Similarly, all energy healing modalities and systems present their respective ontologies and corresponding methodologies, but in the end the flow of energy is directed and maintained by consciousness. This is a fundamentally different outlook on everything that is, whether inside or outside of currently understood *energy work*. Whatever we do, say, build, create, destroy, allow, deny, or repress – in the end all our activities are means and modes of *modulating consciousness*.

Sure, I can use a Tibetan Singing Bowl to create a frequency, a vibration. Sure, my body, or more correctly, my noosphere, perceives that vibration and modulates my consciousness to allow for, or to effect, healing or discomfort. Similarly, I can use a computer program to generate a certain frequency that, when emitted into the noosphere, modulates my consciousness in such a way that changes are effected on a cellular level. This even holds for so-called physical activities: yes, I can massage a muscle to remove a spasm, but what am I doing here on an energy level?

> *I modulate consciousness to release energy at a certain location in the noosphere.*

∞

Firstly, it is just energy. It is only your consciousness that adds meaning to the information: remember, a cramping muscle and a relaxed muscle encode the same, both are energetic constellations, but with different meanings imbued by the consciousness that generates the noosphere. All energetic constellations per se are thus value-free; none is better than the other. This is an important consideration when you enter energy world with the intention to effect change. One needs to understand that deciding for or against a certain energetic expression or constellation is an expression of value. Ideally, one would want to ensure that does not happen. However, we are empowered with this amazing ability to create intent, which is akin to a command to act in the energy world – the purer and les contaminated this intent is by patterns, fears, anger, filters, values, fickle thought, the stronger it is.

165

One important aspect to remember is that consciousness is always self-referential. This means, in effect, no straight lines. Incidentally, you will rarely see straight lines in Nature either. Why? Because they lead away from the noosphere, they could potentially lead into an endless void or abyss, and that would be the end of it. No, living systems are self-referential, self-incremental, and they are dissipative structures. In this energy world, this translates into:

> *You take up energy, you work with it, and then you need to let it go again. Human consciousness is not doing so well in that regard. We are all energetic hoarders of sorts.*

The only remaining activity for consciousness that is energetically neutral is thus to accumulate knowledge about itself, the soul. All knowledge I have about the world needs to say something about myself, otherwise it is akin to a straight line leading away from yourself; it is *meaningless* knowledge. Once you can travel through the *energy world* unaffected, you are truly free and resting within yourself. Western societies have a problem with this and interpret this as *ego*. Yet, this is *self-care*. This is a crucial difference!

Emotions drive us. The meaning is in the word, *e-motion*: the movement of energy. And yet, if you compare that movement to that of a pendulum, the most stable resting point for the pendulum is exactly at the centre. This is where your soul is, or is meant to be. Anything that moves us, and that we cannot let go of, is akin to somebody holding the pendulum to one side, spending willpower or energy on maintaining the pendulum's location and status quo. Once you let go of the pendulum, it will swing about violently, and you can regularly observe this kind of motion in humans. It leads to all kinds of complications and unceasing levels of resentment, emptiness, despair, loneliness, fear, anxiety, anger, etc.

> *Wouldn't it be nice to just let it all go?*

To shed the skin that is too tight, or those burdens that are too heavy, or those memories that are just too painful, and let it all go is like taking a deep breath. In order to take a new breath, you have to first let go of the old breath filling up your lungs. And although we *know* this, we never follow through in doing it properly. For thousands of years we have been getting pointers from religious books of all flavours, on the art of letting go: put them on the altar and walk away (Christianity); acknowledge the emotion and know that it is just temporary (Buddhism); attempting to cleanse oneself of emotional attachments continually (Islam); or striving for *simchah* by tapping into a force that is higher and bigger than oneself (Kabbalah).

> *Letting go does not involve losing control, it involves knowingly transferring control.*

Sure, you might say, all well and good, but what will it *cost* you to do this? And I would ask something like, what do you need to *let go* of? Most often, letting go feels like losing out, when actually it is just the opposite. Yet, one keeps wondering if something else is better on the other side, right? Turn your eyes inward, it's not about letting go of another person, or the marriage, or anything specific in the outside world. Let go of stuff inside! Such as feelings of fear, anger, loneliness, hopelessness, despair, anxiety, or depression. You might say, ok, but I am really scared to let my guard down, I have been disappointed so often in my life, I could not possibly do that! I am worried that if I relax, I get attached to people, circumstances or things again, and I know myself, I will yet again become extremely anxious. In the end, I don't want to feel needy and weak.

When you find your spiritual and emotional centre of *who you are*, a steady stream of endless power flows from it; in order to have a good connection to the Divine, you need a good connection to yourself. Combining your intellect with your gut feeling is like running on turbo all the time; whether it's in the private or the business field, stay connected to yourself. If anything or anybody comes and disconnects you from yourself, take a step back, take a timeout, and reconnect with yourself; that is the only true duty you as a soul have in this life. The stronger your connection with yourself becomes, the less you will be needy and weak. When you trust and love yourself you will walk and talk your truth and not be weak, simply because you will be in your truth all the time. Staying in your truth makes you truly invincible.

Until you stand in your truth, every relationship, whether it is your current one, the next one, or any future one, will reflect you not being in your truth. You will see anger, anxiety, fear, disappointment, resentment, betrayal, but of course also joy and happiness – it will be as if the other person, your partner, will act like a mirror to you. And hence, whenever a relationship fails, *it is never about the other person*. Once you learn about your own truths, and you start heeding and living your truths, outside factors, people, conditions, and situations suddenly lose their power over you. It is like magic.

> *Often we lose perspective, and while we battle ourselves through self-doubt, others might see us in a totally different light, and they might feel intimated by the power we don't live, our potential.*

Human development is fascinating. Not only do innumerable chemical processes and changes take place, but also a multitude of processes and changes in the mental spheres. What makes these processes and changes even more *divine* is that there seems to be no direct correlation between the physical and the mental. Human development thus seems to be twofold and dichotomous rather than unitary and unequivocal. Yet the dichotomy between the physical and the mental is not as strong as it seems to be. It is, rather, apparent that the *symbiotic* relationship between these two entities makes the human being an *apparatus* of great adaptability, sovereignty and, strangely enough, unique unity.

The search for identity is a lifelong quest, and the development of the personality actually encompasses the entire spectrum of human functioning, whether it be intellectual, emotional, social, cognitive, moral, or behavioural. Though various opposing opinions exist about what constitutes *personality*, it would be best if one were to integrate the different views into an overall, conceptually more integrating and holistic approach to the human being and what makes each one of us so special.

Physical and physiological changes an individual undergoes during development always cause psychological changes within the individual. In order to integrate the change of the body with their psychological functioning: how they see themselves, how they perceive others, or how they accommodate sexuality, the individual will find him or herself in a period of distress. Ultimately, the individual can evolve out of this period as a morally stronger, more highly developed, personality.

The search for *identity* is a dynamic organisation of abilities, beliefs, drives, and individual history which the individual self-organises and maintains. In order to obtain and maintain an identity, the person has to identify certain key concepts, patterns of interaction, lifestyles, the value of their own existence, social status, readiness of acceptance, or degrees of intimacy. Identity is an offspring of reality, however subjective that reality might be in the end. The individual identifies his or her unique way of seeing this world, interpreting it, and relating it to significant others. This is normally a lifelong process.

The first major identity crisis was during toddlerhood and childhood, the second one happens during adolescence, and the third one happens during midlife, the midlife crisis: it is always a re-evaluation of the current status quo, of how things are, how they could have been, and how they should have been. The adult, by then, should have enough coping resources, and cognitive and emotional abilities, to constructively change his or her view about everything that matters. Sometimes this is impossible, especially when there lies a generation ahead, and at least one generation behind one's own social, historical position. Wherever you are in life, this is your last position of error so to speak. At any given moment you represent the history of your beingness in this world. It represents the totality of your experiences and internal and external processes that shaped you.

As life progresses through different stages, several things change: the circumstances of life and living; the interpretation of reality and the way of reacting towards perceived stimuli (apart from the primary reaction tendency); the nature, extent and directedness of stressors; the cognitive and emotional coping resources of the individual; and lastly physical and maturational changes in the individual. The interplay between factors in these categories will determine the characteristic extent of the search for self-identity. Another function of self-identity is the achieved stability and ability to *persist* over time. The concept of the *Self* will help to give directedness and validity to the way the individual perceives and integrates stimuli from the environment.

∞

Your island is thus not something that is present overnight, only requiring some tweaks. On the contrary, it is a lifelong project of *becoming*. You may be subject to, or prefer, much tumultuous shaping and redesigning. However, in the end, your life as an island amongst other islands, in a sheer endless sea of energy, is your journey – a spiritual journey in the search for *self-identity*. This is at least as dynamic as life itself.

As much as early human development is dependent on a physical environment that nurtures the organism into growth, at some stage you may have developed sufficient meta-memory to allow you to cease that dependency, and you will be able to feel and think independently of the shape of your island. This is the stage where higher dimensions come into play: the experiences you have as an island do not define you, they just shape the island. Although there is a very intimate link between the shape of your island and the emotional quality of your island, you are more than just that singular island. You will come to realise that your island is just a physical manifestation of a mode of *being* that is an expression of consciousness, energy, and vibration. Whenever you are ready to do so, you will find the courage, the opportunity, and the strength to visit and revisit all your island treasures: its abysses, grottos, dark corners, jungles, pristine landscapes, beaches, cliffs, and mountain tops. And ideally, you will come to realise that they are just experiences, and the question '*Who am I?*' will transcend those experiences, emotions, fears, angers, and loneliness and open up an inner world of great light, strength, and beauty.

Whichever circumstances or constellations you find yourself in, understand that it is just a stage. Allow the stage to pass by letting go of the suffering. Learn what you can from the circumstances, and move on. Moving on does not mean leaving the circumstances, it just means that you are willing to change, that you are willing to let go of how things should be in your mind. If you are bothered by the forest animals in your jungle, you cannot replace them with animals from the mountain areas. Everything in and about your island is in a cyclical relationship with its immediate, smaller and larger environments. Most of these cycles we don't see, feel, hear, smell or taste. We read about them in books, and they get all kinds of fancy labels to denote they are *effects*, something extraordinary, tantamount to a *miracle*. Such effects show us that there are bigger cycles at play; although we can build mind-boggling skyscrapers, we are still embedded in nature, and our developments on a small and in large scale, as individual and as society, are natural processes.

Understand that your island is your sovereign land, no matter what others are saying or doing. When you subscribe to the Divine, only good can come from your actions, and it is in your own best and higher interest to be intimately familiar with your own island. Whichever form or shape your island takes, there is a history of experiences, emotions, and thought processes behind it. Many of those will be below your awareness threshold, but you cannot really claim ignorance of them. Own those too, not just the beautiful beaches or breath taking landscapes of your island; own it all.

Once you do, you will realise that there is even more to realise, to learn, to perceive, and to own. And you keep growing, you open up to new possibilities, you continue your journey. The Divine is literally waiting on you to start exploring, and by the time you have explored your inner worlds, you will turn your eyes even more *in*ward, and find *in* the island what you have been seeking *on* the island.

It thus occurs that while children are afraid of the dark,
adults are afraid of the light. (Plato)

∞

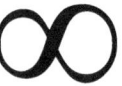

NOOMON XII

∞

FEEL. THINK. LIVE

Over the previous chapters we have been moving from a very physical, intricate, dense, and complex world to a much more translucent, energetic, light, feathery and fantastic one that is not rooted in biology, but in Spirit. Many trendy temporary gurus posit consciousness as being *in* matter; understand, that this is a rather materialist point of view. Instead, the notion that all matter is *of* consciousness would be much more applicable. This is a fundamental and decisive difference. Biology is thus the specific form that a specific embodiment of Spirit takes. That needs to be understood and honoured.

When it comes to healing, this view has significant consequences. Our energy body comes first. Always. It is the link to the energy world and the Divine. When we speak of health, we normally speak of physical, emotional, or mental health. Little do we know about what we need, want, or lack energetically. Our focus on the explicitly physical often brings us to the borders of our belief system, and we find it impossible that a situation, an emotion, a mental state or a physical ailment can disappear within seconds or minutes after we address the energy body. After all, we might have been living with the issue for too long, or the experience or emotion was too hard, or the illness may present itself with way too many symptoms to even consider that all this may vanish like a genie in a bottle – not to speak of the years of suffering we may have had to endure.

Forget all that.

Energy needs to flow, in and out of our systems, towards and away from us. In the physical form, we have our skin to separate us from the outside world. We use our skin as our border, and we repeatedly fail to do so successfully. Hordes of somatic practitioners and therapists will attest to that. Instead, we modulate our experiences in such a way that we can somehow live with them rather than letting them go. Living with them means we store them somewhere in our field of consciousness, be it in the fascia, in our minds, or hearts, or our nervous system(s).

We come from a state of oneness, and we struggle at recreating that oneness because we focus almost exclusively on the physicality of our experiences. And yet we increasingly accept that everything is energy. However, we don't live this:

Suppose you felt an emotion of 'I want xyz', then you would probably go out and buy the physical embodiment of an energy, provided you have the money for that (which is yet another form of energy that you don't have enough of). Your energy body is expressing a need or a blockage, and you would try and fix it with a physical form. Does it work? Look around you, how many physical objects does your household contain?

It would help to see yourself as two entities, where the obvious one is a physical correlation of your energetic one. Provide and give your energetic being, in energetic form, what you would give your physical being in physical form. Providing yourself with whatever you need in energetic form has got nothing to do with selfishness or ego. There is plenty of energy everywhere to provide everybody with all the power and energy and wants and haves that all of us require energetically. It is, in fact, a way of living your truth. So, maybe you do not need the physical hilltop mansion, but you might need the energy of a hilltop mansion. And perhaps you also do not need the physical ten million dollars, but you might need the equivalent energy.

Learn to give to your energy body whatever it needs energetically.

It may not find a physical correspondence, but it will make you feel better about yourself. Why would you want to deprive yourself of energy while gobbling up all the physical stuff you can put your hands on? That just doesn't make sense. You are tasked to find what brings you closer towards your state of flow. No amount of reversal, undoing, turning back the clock, or any other form of negation will align your energies and your physical body to a state where you are a truly dissipative system. Not learning about our true energetic nature, we fail to learn how to deal with energies.

Countless millions, if not billions, of people suffer from the consequences of not knowing how to deal with energy and consciousness; the effect of this is visible in the statistics of any national healthcare system. How can this be? Why is the world so much in a constant state of being mugged?

What is causing this?

The answer lies in our development on Earth. The past millennia have caused our brain to become the strongest muscle in the body, yet it should be our heart, our feelings, our manner of joining intent and action. Energy has the tendency to always teach our consciousness more than we could have anticipated. Consciousness does not grow by knowledge about the world, but by knowledge about ourselves. And when we let our heart centre run, it takes us to the fringes of our own belief system. The halo of the bulb in the dark room does not grow by an analysis of dark and light, but by trusting and believing that beyond the border lies more. In order to achieve that we need a muscle that is not attached to our five senses.

When we replace *analysis* with *discernment*, and *trusting the known* with *trusting the unknown*, we may call it whatever human societies come up with as a label, yet the simple mechanism remains:

> *Healing is a dimension we need to create because it is always other than we thought it was in the first place.*

Why is this? This doesn't make sense, right? Suppose you have illness and you are looking to heal it. You have been to countless doctors, therapists, practitioners, up and down the catalogue of modalities and interventions, the one more illustrious that the other. Yet nothing has changed your condition. You have an image of how a healed body or condition would look and feel, and this image is still within your phenomenological reach. Yet, if I were to ask you to make a

177

drawing of a truly alien being, all you would do is to make a drawing of elements of your consciousness here on this planet, of your life, from your pool of experiences, with a dash of outrageous creativity, and yet it would contain elements of this life, this earth, this incarnation. As fantastical as the creature of your drawing could be, it would still be constituted of this reality's content. *Healing* would be outside your phenomenology.

> *What if healing was more, or better, or more extraordinary, more joyful, more blissful, more everything than you could ever have anticipated, imagined, law-of-attraction-ed, or resonated?*
>
> *We find this so much out of our reach, that we ascribe Divine intervention to the act or the state of absolute healing.*

The first step towards healing is to live your truth. Open your chakras constructively, work on your energetic Self as you would work on your physical Self. Before you give yourself a physical something, give it to yourself energetically first. After you have done so, see whether you still want or need it so badly on the physical level. The way to do this is by means of self-care. The physical world is finite, the energy world is endless. Tap into that resource and give your energetic self what it needs to feel better. Move your centre of consciousness from your brain into your heart, and create healing for yourself from your heart chakra.

> *But what about gratitude?*

Gratitude does not answer the needs of your energy body. Gratitude is a response to the embodiment of an energetic need on the physical plane. There is nothing wrong with being grateful for the little you may have on the physical plane, but allowing your energy body to have its needs satisfied on the energetic level will make you *more* happy, *more* content, *more* at peace, *more* in the flow with the ebb and tide of the waters around your island.

And yet, gratitude is much more than that. It is your level of discernment that you are embedded in a truly gargantuan web of providence where everything has its place and time while nothing and nobody gets lost. It can only be ascribed to human grandeur to believe that free will is not the explicit attempt to diminish the one or other light. What do *you* choose?

> *Claim your right to the energy world around you, and always consider that the perceived physical lack is actually an energetic lack.*

∞

How can one go about doing this? First of all, stop focusing on the bad. If you believe that removing the bad experiences or emotions from your past, by whichever modality, talks to you, you will find a bottomless pit. And often, people just cannot find anything negative having happened in their lives that would explain a present problem or issue. Sometimes people lack love, strength, fortitude, luck, belief, greatness, or countless other emotions or mindsets. No specific experience in their lives actually created the belief system that makes them doubt themselves. It is what it is. Trying to dig in the past is actually not helpful at all, but bringing that energy of greatness, the energy of love, the energy of strength, or any other positive emotions or mindset into one's field of consciousness will tip the scales. Perhaps those emotions are already in the field of consciousness, but one may have pulled up a shield to protect oneself against them (for whatever reason), so they will not be able to be closer than, say, a metre...

Practise looking at yourself with energy eyes. Where do you feel the lack of something, and if you believe you have a protective shield, where do you feel that? And if you were to allow just a pinhead of that desired energy to penetrate that shield of yours, where would you feel that? And once you felt it, where would that energy want to go to? Remember, as a dissipative structure, you need to let that energy out again. Create a circular system, in on the one side, and out somewhere else. That will create a drag and pull in more of the same energy. And suddenly, we find ourselves back in the vicinity of the Law of Attraction. However here is the fundamental difference:

> *To get through the night, you need to become the night.*

179

What does this actually mean??

The more you become like water, the less you will resist water. The more you become like Light, the less you will resist the Light. The more you allow your own Higher Self and energy, the less you will be affected by that of others. Or, put differently: You cannot vibrate higher if your need for higher vibration is not met on an energetic level.

Where you resist your own energy flows, you will generate emotions: anger, sadness, despair, depression, untruths, loneliness, hatred, frustration, and jealousy. The bandwidth of human emotions – and thus human suffering – is almost endless. Allowing your own energy and *answering your energetic needs with energetic answers* allows you to love yourself, to live your truths, and to be content with how, what, when, and where you are. It also allows you to answer physical, emotional, intellectual and spiritual demands differently, if they appear in your life then.

Sounds like paradise to me....

Consider the notion that for a dissipative structure such as a human being, at the base of all physical symptoms lies a disruption of energetic flow. Surely not all symptoms can be reduced to a disruption in the energy system, right? When the human genome was mapped over the past decades, the researchers found that we had way too few genes to explain all the proteins in our bodies. In addition, there were living organisms with more and fewer genes than ourselves, and less expression of genetic features than we do. This disconnect gave rise to what is now called epigenetics – the notion that our perception of reality somehow affects the expression of our genes.

However, why would organisms develop such a feature? Surely not for survival; it is easier to fine-tune the existing processes of reproduction and, say, lay a million more eggs, than to go through trial and error and epigenetically switch on or off one or more genes of a pool of hundreds or thousands. If we approach the discussion from the angle of consciousness, things change dramatically.

Where consciousness is the only tool you have in the energy world, attention is what consciousness does in the energy world.

Practise the flow of energy into, around, and out of your body and field of consciousness, and do that for each and every other positive aspect of your *Self* that you believe you are lacking. If you say that you are lacking self-confidence, why probe in your past instead of allowing the energy of that to flow through your energetic system? You probably block all incoming energy that brings to you that feeling and understanding of self-confidence, yet you crave and hunger for it all the time. This one blockage that you might need to overcome may be the reason for your current incarnation. Don't ruin it (again).

If you allow the energy in, it always addresses a positive aspect of your being. Practice on a daily basis because it will stimulate a circulation of energy that will become so strong that it pulls in even more energy. Once you have outgrown your limitations and the energies are freely flowing, gratitude will come all by itself because you will feel saturated.

We humans have many such blockages. Most of them are there for a reason, namely to protect us from energy of others or the outside world. As ridiculous as some may find the concept of energy, we all act according to our sense of energy. In a universe of energy, such blockages or shields make perfect sense. And they are manageable by consciousness, as is everything else that is of energy. Where energy condenses into what we call matter, it is a bit more complicated to change and manipulate – for that you have a physical body.

How many of your apparent physical problems and constellations in life are actually based on energetic constellations and your shield against the flow of energy?

Understand that it is your right, and prerogative, to do and be as you wish. Even though you have an energy body, your injuries - and your blockages - form part of your journey towards understanding. Throwing phrases like 'you have to let go', 'you need to forgive', or 'you need to raise your vibration' and other New Age terms at you will just add insult to injury. Your shields and your blockages are there *for* you, not *against* you – even though it may feel like it. In fact, your systems are working perfectly well most of the times in protecting you. Who is any person, or any therapist, to say that you need to do, act, think, or be otherwise? Forgiveness will only happen when you have managed to step *out* of your pain. Until that one singular moment where and when you do, any talk about forgiveness is futile. Yes, you may have read many books on the subject, but understand that all you ever do is modulate your consciousness towards inclusion of all, towards dissolution of all borders, boundaries, shields and blockages.

> *Healing is a dimension we create! Use whatever you have. Start wherever you are in life. Don't wait for an apparently right condition or circumstance.*

> *Be now! Do now!*

So *en*lightened, you will be able and empowered to *en*gage with the world differently. Heal where you go, heal whomever you meet. Meet yourself regularly. Sensitise yourself to the energetic reality of life. Observer yourself when you meet somebody: your hands, your eyes, your ears, or your sense of smell – they all go where energy goes. Look at the gestures of another person, and you will realise they are painting energy in mid-air. This is where it happens; they are actually putting their hand(s) right on the spot. You might not experience it like that, but with a little practise and listening to your sixth sense, you will realise that subconsciously you may already be subscribing to this invisible world, even though consciously you might subscribe to a full-blown material world.

> *Understand that when you marry these two dimensions, new pathways will emerge that take you towards more wonders and mysteries – the deeper you look, the bigger the mystery.*

From previous chapters you will remember the discussion about belief systems – the boundaries of these are normally defined by an energetic shield, wall, or blockage. If you have a belief system about yourself that you are not worthy of being loved, you will block such energy from reaching you even if you have the most loving partner telling and showing you right in front of you. It may feel like a disconnect to you, and people often refer to an invisible wall between them and others and the world, or there is a wall right in front of their face, their chest, around their body, their hands are covered in a disconnecting clay, etc. The possibilities for how people refer to these invisible separations are almost endless, and despite them being invisible, almost everybody has such an image of himself or herself at some stage in life.

Why do we refer to ourselves in energy terms? Where does this come from? And why do we keep ignoring this?

We are constantly making judgement calls. Every day, if we need to choose between left or right, option A or option B, we make a judgement – and judgements create shields, walls, and blockages. Judgements enable you to protect yourself, albeit at the price of losing connection. This happens in the physical world as much as in the energy world. We need to deal with energy differently than we currently do if we want to reverse our wiring for protection to a wiring for connection. The fact that you like the colour blue more than the colour red, or you prefer one taste to another taste, or one pattern to another pattern, is an indication of your energetic constellation. Inherently, it is also telling about your limitations, your world views, your blockages, walls and shields. An experienced energy practitioner can read you in a split-second; unlike the physical world, in the energy world there are no secrets. That really is not as threatening as you might think it is (if you feel antagonised now, check where that energy is sitting in or around your body and try to channel it towards the edge of your physical body so it can leave your field), because there are no good or bad colours, only colours, and there is no good or bad energy, just energy.

Whether anything is perceived as good or bad is exclusively the making of your consciousness.

When you reject something that is, say, orange, you might end up rejecting an orange sunset, an orange animal, a person with orange hair, orange fruit, etc. The result of this is that your energy body is starved of the *energy of orange*. Consequently, you may experience all kinds of energetic cravings cloaked as physical cravings. For example, you might gobble up orange crisps while developing a wall that prevents you from realising that the orange crisps are extremely unhealthy, and that they are actually orange, and suddenly you find yourself not being able to lose weight despite doing everything in your power (literally) to get rid of excess weight. A few years down the line, you might experience additional health issues due to those pesky orange-coloured crisps that taste sensational, yet orange.

If this sounds familiar to you, try to give yourself the energy of orange, see where your wall is, how it feels, and how you are actually blocking energy instead of letting it flow through you. Find the entry point of that energy, and find the exit point of that energy. Once you do that, you have mapped a new pathway for that kind of energy, and you are safe to lower your wall or let go of that blockage because you now know how to deal with the energy; being a dissipative structure is the healthy and above all natural state of your consciousness.

Unlearn the confines of physical reality!

Unlike many religious traditions, getting to know the energy world is not like using an algorithm that locks you on an idealistic path, running sequential instructions until the ideal state is achieved. While it may help many to deal with the onslaught of physical reality on their consciousness and energy system, you are tasked with removing internal barriers. This is arduous for many, impossible for many more, and quite easy for only a few. But rest assured that you don't need to improve yourself all the time as if you are ticking off milestones. Rather, just be.

Be within as without, and by being you are doing, despite not focusing on doing anything except being...

This kind of healing is free of charge. It is provided as part of this universe and your existence. Don't believe me, or any other person who is telling you or writing about this. Go and find out for yourself. The truth needs no bearer, guru, carrier, or defender. The truth is there to be found by anybody who is eager to seek it. Whether you do, or not, is the contextual framework of your existence. And you are free to do it, or not, without the sword of any form of reprimand hovering above your head. Such is the grace of the Divine, and to experience life is an absolute blessing.

> *You are tasked to open up yourself to such energies, to allow yourself to be reminded by everything you encounter in life of your divine origin. All of what you call life is there to help you. Take that step forward, allow yourself to be amazed, to be taught, to learn and accept, and all else will follow.*

When you embark on this path, you will come to realise that the concept of cognition we spoke about in earlier chapters has changed to a more enlightened cognition, enriched by energy, enriched by a humility that is rooted in Spirit. It will allow you to be *in* this world and less *of* this world (you will find numerous passages about this in religious texts). The repercussions of your changed cognition and consciousness will ripple through your entire life. When you attend to your own walls, blockages and shields, your enlightened consciousness will also ripple to others around you. Something happens when you allow yourself to work with energy consciously – it is as if it carries information. Energy is understood by every person, every animal, every plant and every living organism. It is the universal language we tried to recreate in Babel.

> *Let your enlightenment be like a virus spreading change and healing throughout the world. You need not declare yourself a healer or a teacher. In fact, you will abstain from doing so because your need to translate your Self and your soul into a language you believe the other person can understand simply falls away.*

185

When you add the repertoire of energy language to your field of consciousness, you open yourself up to learning just by allowing the energy of an object to enter your space, flow through you, and out again. This is a transformational, almost alchemic process of being in the world. There are just four simple steps to doing this:

- *Allow the energy to enter your space. See where it enters your field.*

- *Will it to flow out of your body again.*

- *Observe where it flows to and how it exits your body and field again.*

- *If it feels stuck (e.g. in your throat or stomach), will it to flow away from that area and find an exit point.*

Do this with everything. Take a rock and initiate the energy transfer. Take gemstones, objects, plants, animals, and do the same thing. Learn to be dissipative: allow, resolve blockages, walls, and shields, will the energy to move out again, follow the energy, allow it to leave again. The result of this is that you act like a toroidal structure, creating an energetic suction that will persist unless you tinker with the dissipation of energy. You can then allow some things, people, and animals more than others. The ensuing enrichment of your life is beyond your wildest dreams.

Similarly, you can come into *the knowing* of everything else in the world. Take the book you bought yesterday and have not started yet. Take in the energy of that, see where it enters, where it sits, and how it leaves your system again. If you then proceed to read the book word by word with your left brain, you will find that, uncannily, you know the content already. When your consciousness focuses on energy, you will find that you rely increasingly less on your actual physical eyes.

> *And then you go out, and you learn from all of Creation. When you allow this, energy and information becomes interchangeable. And by doing that, you actually learn all about yourself. This is what reality is there for.*

When you learn to allow yourself to operate as intended, unconditional love is a structural coupling of your consciousness to the rest of the field of consciousness and energy. It is a direct consequence of energy work, but it is extremely difficult for people that are stuck in, say, pain or hatred. How could I possibly forgive my attacker of twenty years ago, when I have been living with that pain and despair for so long that I cannot even imagine how it feels not to have these emotions anymore? Understand that what you need is not more protection, more barriers, more blockages, more vigilance, but rather more information, more trust, more energy, more love. And the way to bring this into your life is via the energy route!

The secret here is not to hoard energy like money in the bank, but to give it all away by letting it go. The secret lies not in how elaborate your blockage, your wall, your shield or protection is, but to open up to all forms of energy. It is your walls, your blockages, and your protection that create judgment. This is what makes you feel emotions. The goal is not an emotionless state, but the ability to let all the energies go again.

Remain dissipative.

How does a crying child make you feel? Where do you feel it? Let the energy flow, let it pass through you. If you don't, you will become distressed. The same goes for all other forms of energy, whether they appear to you incarnated as an animal, as a tree, a rock, the abusive partner, the taxi, or the robot. However, no matter how intentionally you allow the energy of others to flow through you, the other person might not want to change or heal right now. For example, it is the prerogative of the abusive partner to stay abusive. It does not mean that you need to endure the abuse despite your best attempts at healing yourself. In fact, staying in the abusive relationship is a sure indication that you have not healed (yet).

For those of us who are not in such a relationship, give yourself the energy of an abusive relationship. See where you feel it, if at all. If you don't, you have protection. Try to lower that shield and feel the energy, then find a pathway for its release. That will be your process of healing yourself. Do this with everything you eat, drink, hear, see, contemplate, read, experience, smell, or feel.

> *Heal yourself. Do it right away. Change your incarnation, and change that of those you touch. Heal the world. You don't have to solve the problems, just help them along, help them evolve.*

∞

The mindset makes or breaks the Healer, not the techniques. Healing happens when consciousness changes. There is nothing I can do to another person in terms of healing. I can bring my level of consciousness into the proximity of theirs, and when they at least partially resonate with it, they will change their consciousness; and then healing happens as a by-product. Even if I use a physical intervention, it is actually just my different kind of consciousness that interacts with the other consciousness: here, try this change! When there is a pathway, the client consciousness changes in response to changed awareness, as it comes in contact with mine; and then the intervention works. With others, the intervention won't work, or nothing works. All healing is a dimension we create by changing consciousness. It is more than just programming that cloaks our belief systems. Healing is resonance with a different state of consciousness.

> *When you are ready to do this, you will realise that the 'who am I?' of the previous chapters is not to find your calling, the truth, or even enlightenment. It is a question that is to dissolve you, the questioner, beyond all words, pictures, and symbolism.*

Several modulators influence our tuning into one of many realities: our five senses, our gut feeling, extrasensory perception, emotions, thought processes, and what we call reality. The bodily link to *this* apparent reality is so strong, that for most people only hallucinogens can break the causal link. The million-dollar question is: how do we entrain the brain to a different reality? How can brain waves and synchronization be modified? Many methods have been tried already, and for some they work better than for others.

Nevertheless, like objects and organisms, words are also antennas. The word 'love' represents a different design than the word of 'anger'. Observe which words you surround yourself with, and which words you use to express energetic experience. Similarly, observe which kind of frequencies you consume all day, every day, all year, and every year, for decades or lifetimes. What are the determinants in terms of frequency and vibration, and how do these influence your life? See how your ecosystem of antenna designs expresses or collides with your inner truths, your belief system, and your relationship with the Divine. How many of your struggles and battles could possibly stem from this? Find out, this is your life. Your reality is actually a plethora of vibrational properties of various antenna designs such as objects, words, or people. Give yourself the energies you need, even if that means changing your life from head to toe, simply because even if there is nothing to believe in, always believe in your own soul. It is your core vibration, the one that forges your multidimensional metaphysical existence.

Heal that above all else! Be brave. Fear nothing!

The impact of a different epistemological approach can be shown in a discussion about quantum mechanics. The contemporary marriage of quantum mechanics and spirituality has a serious drawback, which is commonly referred to as *Many Worlds*. Firstly, when the wave function refers to multiple superimposed states of reality that collapse as soon as measured, the implication is that there are multiple realities that might as well be aspects of (probably) one ontological reality. In spirituality, this ontological reality is referred to as *Oneness*. Sounds good, but is this correct? Secondly, at every moment of our lives where we create a wave function collapse, reality splits into the one we continue in, and those we didn't. This approach results in an incomprehensible multitude of not just particles, but entire worlds or universes, and all this for only one observer. The problem grows exponentially as we add more observers and measurements. In addition, this approach requires a birds-eye, or even a higher order view of all. However, can we really do this? If our every act of observation creates a reality, how could we ever take an overall view of Oneness? The multiple worlds argument is haphazardly used and sold in the industry of modern spirituality.

However, despite this gross, incomprehensible vastness of multiple worlds, what explanatory value does this approach have once we discount the staggering superfluity of worlds? More often than not, it leads people to envision, to dream, to resonate, to vibrate, to quantum jump, or to do all kinds of activities just to be taken away from *now* to a position of attempting to self-improve continually.

Let's try a different approach that is based on what was discussed in this book. When we say that my observation collapsed the wave function, I am back to the old notion of myself acting in an objective reality, which is not objective until I measure it. However, if the notion of an objective reality is a fallacy, then the collapsing wave function doesn't say anything about the particle, but rather something about myself, the observer. Which reality the wave function collapses into is an expression of my consciousness, not an aspect of a primary reality.

I wish you safe travels through any and all of your dimensions.

Create wisely, and witness Creation.

Be gentle and compassionate to all Living.

Be humble and grateful.

Feel. Think. Live.

Disclaimer:

As you increasingly allow the Divine Light into your life, above will happen automatically.

There is nothing you need to do, except to allow the Light. It will grow on you.

And thus I wish you well on your paths through your lives.

∞

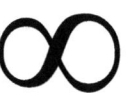

FURTHER READING

Al-Hussaini, A., Dorvlo, A., & Antony, S. (2001). Vipassana meditation: A naturalistic, preliminary observation in Muscat. *Journal for Scientific Research, Medical Sciences, 3*(2), 87-92.

Atkin, A. (2007). *Does All Begin with Consciousness? (Some theoretical speculations).* Lincoln, Nebraska, USA: iUniverse, Inc.

Baird, J. D. (2015). *Epigenetics and Well-Being.* Retrieved from World of Psychology: http://psychcentral.com/blog/archives/2015/07/11/epigenetics-and-well-being/

Barabási, A.-L. (2002). *Linked: The New Science of Networks.* Cambridge, Massachuesetts, USA: Perseus.

Bengston, W. (n.d.). *A non-invasive, information-based healing method.* Retrieved from Bengston Research: http://www.bengstonresearch.com

Bethrick, D. (n.d.). *Examining CARM's "Entropy Argument".* Retrieved from Katholon - Rational Thinking for the 21st Century: http://katholon.com/CARM/Entropy.htm

Bohm, D. (1993). *The Undivided Universe: An Ontological Interpretation of Quantum Theory.* London: Routledge.

Breathnach, S. B. (2000). *Somehing More: excavating your authentic self.* New York: Grand Central Publishing.

Brennan, B. A. (1988). *Hands of Light - A Guide to Healing Through the Human Energy Field.* New York: Bantam Books.

Brosnan, C. (2016, May 3). Epistemic cultures in complementary medicine: knowledge-making in university departments of

osteopathy and Chinese medicine. *Health Sociology Review,*
25(2), 171-186. doi:10.1080/14461242.2016.1171161

Buchanan, B., & Shortliffe, E. H. (1984). *Rule-Based Expert Systems.*
Reading, Massachusetts, USA: Addison-Wesley.

Buchanan, M. (2002). *Small World: Uncovering Nature's Hidden*
Networks. London: Weidenfeld and Nicolson.

Capra, F. (1996). *The Web of Life.* London: HarperCollins.

Capra, F. (2002). *The Hidden Connections - A Science for Sustainable*
Living. USA: First Anchor Books.

Carnap, R. (1994). *An Introduction to The Philosophy of Science.* New
York: Basic Books.

Chalmers, A. (1999). *What is This Thing Called Science?* (3rd ed.). St.
Lucia: University of Queensland Press.

Chia, M. (2007). *Fusion of the Five Elements.* Rochester: Destiny
Books.

Chia, M. (2008). *Healing Light of the Tao.* Rochester: Destiny Books.

Church of Spiritual Science. (n.d.). Retrieved from
http://www.churchofspiritualscience.org/index.html

Corbin, H. (1998). *Alone with the Alone: Creative Imagination in the*
Sūfism of Ibn 'Arabī: Creative Imagination in the Sufism of Ibn
'Arabi. Princeton: Princeton University Press.

Davenport, T. H., & Prusak, L. (2000). *Working Knowledge: How*
Organisations Manage What They Know. Boston: Harvard
Business School Press.

de Chardin, P. T. (1959, reprint 2002). *The Phenomenon of Man.* New
York, USA: Harper Perennial.

Dempster, B. (n.d.). Sympoietic and Autopoietic Systems: A New
Distinction for Self-Organizing Systems. Waterloo,
Ontario, Canada: University of Waterloo.

Dennett, D. C. (2017). *From Bacteria to Bach and Back: The Evolution of*
Minds. New York: W. W. Norton & Company.

Dennett, D. C. (Reprint 1996). *Darwin's Dangerous Idea: Evolution and the Meanings of Life.* New York, USA: Simon & Schuster.

Dispenza, J. (2014). *You Are The Placebo.* London: Hay House.

Dixon, N. (2000). *Common Knowledge.* Boston: Harvard Busines School Press.

Dole, G. F. (2018). *The Universe and I: Where Science & Spirituality Meet.* West Chester: Swedenborg Foundation.

Dougans, I. (2005). *Reflexology - The 5 Elements and their 12 Meridians: A Unique Approach.* Thorsons Element.

Doyle, J. (1984). Expert Systems Without Computers or Theory and Trust in Artificial Intelligence. *AI Magazine, 5*(2), 59-63.

Dresser, H. W. (1921). *The Quimby Manuscripts.* Thomas Y. Crowell Co.

Dreyfus, H. L. (1992). *What Computers Still Can't Do: A Critique of Artificial Reason.* Cambridge, Massachusetts, USA: MIT Press.

Duda, R. O., & Shortliffe, E. H. (1983, April 15). Expert Systems Research. *Science, 220*(4594), 261-268.

Etxeberria, A. (2004). Autopoiesis and Natural Drift: Genetic Information, Reproduction and Evolution Revisited. *Artificial Life, 10*(3), 347-360. Retrieved from http://www.ehu.eus/ias-research/doc/2004_etxe_ALife.pdf

Fidelibus, J. (1996). *Postmodernism and You: Psychology.* Retrieved from Xenos Christian Fellowship: http://www.xenos.org/ministries/crossroads/dotpsy.htm

Fisher, J. (1984). *The Case for Reincarnation.* Toronto: Collins.

Fleischaker, G. R. (1992). Questions concerning the ontology of autopoiesis and the limits of its utility. *International Journal of General Systems, 21*(2), 131-141. Retrieved from http://www.univie.ac.at/constructivism/archive/fulltexts/2682.html

Forbes, D., & Higgins, R. (2005). *Human Pin Code.* Johannesburg: eB&W Publishers Ltd.

Forrest, C. B. (2014, February). A Living Systems Perspective on Health. *Medical Hypotheses, 82*(2), 209-214. doi:http://dx.doi.org/10.1016/j.mehy.2013.11.040

Freemantle, F., & Chogyam, T. (1987). *The Tibetan Book of the Dead.* London: Shambhala.

Giddens, A. (1991). *Modernity and Self-Identity.* Oxford: Blackwell Publishing.

Gladwell, M. (2002). *The Tipping Point: How Little Things Can Make A Big Difference.* New York, USA: Little, Brown & Company.

Gleick, J. (1988). *Chaos.* London: Sphere.

Gräff, J., Kim, D., Dobbin, M. M., & Tsai, L.-H. (2011, April 1). Epigenetic Regulation of Gene Expression in Physiological and Pathological Brain Processes. *Physiological Reviews, 91*(2), 603-649. doi:10.1152/physrev.00012.2010

Grazzi, L., d'Amico, D., Raggi, A., Leonardi, M., Ciusani, E., Corsini, E., Sansone, E. (2017, May). Mindfulness and pharmacological prophylaxis have comparable effect on biomarkers of inflammation and clinical indexes in chronic migraine with medication overuse: results at 12 months after withdrawal. *Neurological Science, 38*(1), 173-175. doi:10.1007/s10072-017-2874-0

Green, H. S. (2000). *Information Theory and Quantum Physics : Physical Foundations for Understanding the Conscious Process.* Berlin: Springer-Verlag Berlin and Heidelberg GmbH & Co. KG.

Greenwood, S. (2005). *The Nature of Magic - An Anthropology of Consciousness.* New York, USA: Berg Publishers.

Gunaratne, S. (2007). Systems approaches and communication research: The age of entropy. *Communications, 32*, 79-96.

Gurdjieff, G. I. (1981, reprint). *Life is real only then, when "I am".* New York, USA: Penguin Books Ltd.

Hall, S. (1996). Introduction: Who needs 'Identity'? In S. Hall, & O. du Gay (Eds.), *Questions of Cultural Identity* (pp. 1-17). London: Sage.

Hameroff, S. (2014). Consciousness, Microtubules, & 'Orch OR': A 'Space-time Odyssey'. *Journal of Consciousness Studies, 21*(3-4), pp. 126-153.

Hameroff, S., & Chopra, D. (2012). The "Quantum Soul": A Scientific Hypothesis. In A. Moreira-Almeida, & F. S. Santos (Eds.), *Exploring Frontiers of the Mind-Brain Relationship: Mindfulness in Behavioral Health.* Springer Science+Business Media.

Hayles, N. (1999). *How We Became Posthuman.* Chicago, Illinois, USA: University of Chicago Press.

Hendryx, J. (2014, March). The Bioenergetic Model in Osteopathic Diagnosis and Treatment: An FAAO Thesis, Part 1. *The American Academy of Osteopathy Journal, 24*(1), pp. 12-20. Retrieved from http://files.academyofosteopathy.org/AAOJ/2014/AAOJ_March2014.pdf

Hendryx, J. (2014, June). The Bioenergetic Model in Osteopathic Diagnosis and Treatment: An FAAO Thesis, Part 2. *The American Academy of Osteopathy Journal, 24*(2), pp. 10-20. Retrieved from http://files.academyofosteopathy.org/AAOJ/2014/AAOJ_June2014.pdf

Horscroft, J. A., Kotwica, A. O., Laner, V., West, J. A., Hennis, P. J., Levett, D. Z., Murray, A. J. (2017, May 16). Metabolic basis to Sherpa altitude adaptation. (G. L. Semenza, Ed.) *Proceedings of the National Academy of Sciences of the United States of America.* Retrieved from http://www.pnas.org/content/early/2017/05/16/1700527114.full.pdf

Hunt, T. (2011). Kicking the Psychophysical Laws into Gear: A New Approach to the Combination Problem. *Journal of Consciousness Studies, 18*(11), 96-134. Retrieved from http://www.researchgate.net/publication/263491208_Kicking_the_Psychophysical_Laws_into_Gear_A_New_Approach_to_the_Combination_Problem

Jackson, P. (1998). *Introduction to Expert Systems* (3rd ed.). Addison-Wesley.

Joye, S. R. (2016). The Pribram-Bohm Holoflux Theory of Consciousness: An Integral Interpretation of the Theories of Karl Pribram, David Bohm, and Pierre Teilhard de Chardin. *Ph.D. Dissertation*. San Francisco, California, USA: California Institute of Integral Studies. Retrieved from http://www.heartmath.org/research/research-library/dissertations/pribram-bohm-holoflux-theory-of-consciousness/

Jung, C. (1991). *Psychology and the East*. New York: Ark Paperbacks.

Jung, C. (1993). *Memories, Dreams, Reflections*. London: Fontana.

Kastrup, B. (2018). The Universe in Consciousness. *Journal of Consciousness Studies, 25*(6), 125-155.

Kauffman, S. (1993). *The Origins of Order*. New York: Oxford University Press.

Kessels, J. W. (2002). You cannot be smart against your will. In B. Garvey, & B. Williamson (Eds.), *Beyond Knowledge Management* (pp. 47-52). Harlow: Pearson Education.

Kessels, J. W., & Keursten, P. (2002). The changing relationship between work and learning: Creating a knowledge productive work environment. *Lifelong Learning in Europe, 7*(2), 104-113.

Kirsch, I., & Sapirstein, G. (1998). Listening to Prozac but Hearing Placebo: A Meta-Analysis of Antidepressant Medication. *Prevention & Treatment, 1*. Retrieved from http://psychrights.org/research/Digest/CriticalThinkRxCites/KirschandSapirstein1998.pdf

Kirsch, I., Deacon, B. J., Huedo-Medina, T. B., Scoboria, A., Moore, T. J., & Johnson, B. T. (2008, February 26). Initial Severity and Antidepressant Benefits: A Meta-Analysis of Data Submitted to the Food and Drug Administration. *PLOS Medicine*. doi:http://doi.org/10.1371/journal.pmed.0050045

Kuhn, T. (1962). *The Structure of Scientific Revolutions*. Chicago: University of Chicago Press.

Laszlo, E. (2007). *Science and the Akashic Field: An Integral Theory of Everything* (2nd ed.). Rochester: Inner Traditions.

Lenzo, V., Buccheri, T., Sindorio, C., Belvedere, A., Fries, W., & Quattropani, M. C. (2013). Metacognition and negative emotions in clinical practice. A preliminary study with patients with bowel disorder. *Mediterranean Journal of Clinical Psychology MJCP, 1*(2). doi:10.6092/2282-1619/2013.2.918

Lichtenberg, P., Heresco-Levy, U., & Nitzan, U. (n.d.). The ethics of the placebo in clinical practice. *Journal of Medical Ethics*. doi:http://dx.doi.org/10.1136/jme.2002.002832

Lohrey, A. (2018). *The Evolution of Consciousness: A New Science*. Princeton, New Jersey, USA: ICRL Press.

Loyd, A., & Johnson, B. (2011). *The Healing Code*. London: Hodder & Stoughton.

Luhmann, N. (1995). *Social Systems*. Stanford, California, USA: Stanford University Press.

Malhotra, Y. (2001). Expert Systems for Knowledge Management: Crossing the Chasm between Information Processing and Sense Making. *Expert Systems with Applications, 20*, 7-16.

Martin, H. (1996). *Menschheit auf dem Prüfstand* (2nd ed.). Berlin: Springer Verlag.

Maturana, H., & Varela, F. (1980). *Autopoiesis and Cognition*. Dordrecht, Netherlands.

Maxwell, J. C. (1871, reprint 2001). *Theory of Heat*. New York, USA: Dover Publishing.

Mercier, P. (2009). *The Chakra Bible: The definitive guide to working with chakras.* London: Godsfield Press.

Minsky, M. (1988). *The Society of Mind.* New York: Simon & Schuster.

Minsky, M. (2007). *The Emotion Machine: Commonsense Thinking, Artificial Intelligence, and the Future of the Human Mind.* New York: Simon & Schuster.

Newton, M. (1994). *Jouney of Souls: Case Studies of Life between Lives.* Woodbury: Llewellyn Publications.

Newton, M. (2014). *Destiny of Souls: New Case Studies of Life between Lives.* Woodbury, Minnesota, USA: Llewellyn Publications.

Nicolis, G. (1995). *Introduction to Non-linear Science.* Cambridge: Cambridge University Press.

Nilsson, N. J. (2009). *The Quest for Artificial Intelligence - A History of Ideas and Achievements.* Cambridge University Press.

Nonaka, I., & Takeuchi, H. (1995). *The Knowledge-Creating Company.* New York: Oxford University Press.

Nunez, R. E. (1997). Eating Soup with Chopsticks: Dogmas, Difficulties and Alternatives in the Study of Conscious Experience. *Journal of Consciousness Studies, 4*(2), pp. 143-166.

Ohmae, K. (2005). *The Next Global Stage - Challenges and Opportunities in our Borderless World.* Upper Saddle River, New Jersey, USA: Wharton School Publishing.

Ouspensky, P. D. (1949, reprint). *In Search of the Miraculous.* Brace: Harcourt.

Overbye, D. (2006, March 14). *Far Out, Man. But Is It Quantum Physics?* Retrieved from What the Bleep Do We Know!?: http://www.whatthebleep.com/reviews/03-17-06-nytimes.shtml

Papert, S., & Harel, I. (1991). *Situating Constructionism.* Ablex Publishing Corporation.

Pizzorno, J. E., Murray, M. T., & Joiner-Bey, H. (2008). *The Clinician's Handbook of Natural Medicine* (2nd ed., Vols. Verhandelingen der Koninklijke Nederlandse Akademie van Wetenschappen, Afd. Letterkunde, Nieuwe Reeks). Elsevier Health Sciences.

Popp, F.-A. (1989). *Electromagnetic Bio-information* (2nd ed.). Urban & Schwarzenberg.

Popp, F.-A. (n.d.). *Consciousness as Evolutionary Process based on Coherent States*. Retrieved from International Institute of Biophysics: http://www.lifescientists.de/publication/pub2003-04-11.htm

Popper, K. R. (1999). *The Logic of Scientific Discovery*. New York: Routledge.

Porter, M. E. (1980). *Competitive Strategy*. New York, NY, USA: Free Press.

Prigogine, I., & Stengers, I. (1984). *Order out of Chaos*. London: Heinemann.

Quattropani, M. C., Lenzo, V., Belvedere, A., & Friess, W. (2014). Dysfunctional metacognitive beliefs and gastrointestinal disorders. Beyond an 'organic'/'functional' categorization in the clinical practice. *Mediterranean Journal of Clinical Psychology MJCP, 2*(1). doi:10.6092/2282-1619/2014.2.955

Rabinovitz, A. (n.d.). *Complexity and Entropy: Human Creativity vs. the Heat Death of the Universe*. Retrieved from http://www.pages.nyu.edu/~air1/Complexity%20and%20Entropy.htm

Rajvanshi, A. K. (n.d.). *Cloud computing as a theory of reincarnation*. Retrieved from http://www.nariphaltan.org/cloudcomputing.htm

Resnick, M. (1997). *Turtles, Termites, and Traffic Jams*. Cambridge, Massachuesetts, USA: MIT Press.

Rockart, J. F. (1979, March/April). Chief Executives Define Their Own Information Needs. *Harvard Business Review*.

Romens, S. E., McDonald, J., Svaren, J., & Pollak, S. D. (2015, February 14). Associations between early life stress and gene methylation in children. (C. G. Coll, Ed.) *Child Development, 86*(1), pp. 303–309. Retrieved from http://onlinelibrary.wiley.com/doi/10.1111/cdev.12270/full

Rose, S. (1999). Précis of Lifelines: Biology, freedom, determinism. *Behavirousal and Brain Sciences, 22*(5), 871-921. Retrieved from http://eprints.lse.ac.uk/12103/1/Rose%27s%20homeodynamic%20perspective%20is%20not%20an%20alternative%20to%20Neo-Darwinism(lsero).pdf

Rose, S. (2012, April 16). Genetics, Reductionism and Autopoiesis. Wiley Online Library. doi:10.1002/9780470015902.a0005895.pub2

Rubik, B. (2002, December). The Biofield Hypothesis: Its Biophysical Basis and Role in Medicine. *The Journal of Alternative and Complementary Medicine, 8*(6), 703-717.

Ruiz, D. M. (2018). *The Four Agreements: A Practical Guide to Personal Freedom (A Toltec Wisdom Book)* (10th ed.). San Rafael, California, USA: Amber-Allen Publishing.

Russo, R., Cristiano, C., Avagliano, C., Raso, G. M., Canani, R. B., Meli, R., la Rana, G. (2017, May). Gut-brain Axis: Role of Lipids in the Regulation of Inflammation, Pain and CNS Diseases. *Current Medicinal Chemistry, 24*(42). Retrieved from http://www.eurekaselect.com/150145/article

Schatten, M., & Baca, M. (2008, October 9). A Critical Review of Autopoietic Theory and its Applications To Living, Social, Organizational and Information Systems. *Društvena istraživanja : Journal for General Social Issues*, 837-852. Retrieved 2017, from http://hrcak.srce.hr/60121

Scientific Study of Consciousness-Related Physical Phenomena. (n.d.). Retrieved from Princeton Engineering Anomalies Research: http://www.pearlab.icrl.org/index.html

Shalev, I., Moffitt, T. E., Braithwaite, A. W., Danese, A., Fleming, N. I., Goldman-Mellor, S., Caspi, A. (2014). Internalizing disorders and leukocyte telomere erosion: a prospective study of depression, generalized anxiety disorder and post-traumatic stress disorder. *Molecular Psychiatry, 19*(11), 1163-1170. doi:10.1038/mp.2013.183

Shannon, C. E. (1964). *The Mathematical Theory of Communication.* Urbana, USA: University of Illinois Press.

Stearn, J. (1989). *Edgar Cayce - The Sleeping Prophet.* New York: Bantam Books.

Strogatz, S. (2004). *Sync: How Order Emerges from Chaos in the Universe, Nature, and Daily Life.* New York: Hachette Books.

Sullivan, G. M. (2011). Getting Off the "Gold Standard": Randomized Controlled Trials and Education Research. *Journal of Graduate Medical Education, 3*(3), 285–289. Retrieved from http://doi.org/10.4300/JGME-D-11-00147.1

Szent-Györgyi, A. (1977). Drive in Living Matter to Perfect Itself. *Synthesis 1, 1*(1), 14-26.

Targ, R. (2012). *The Reality of ESP: A Physicist's Proof of Psychic Abilities.* Wheaton: Quest Books.

Taylor, M. (2003). *The Moment of Complexity: Emerging Network Culture.* Chicago, Illinois, USA: University of Chicago Press.

Tegmark, M. (2014). *Our Mathematical Universe: My Quest for the Ultimate Nature of Reality.* New York: Alfred A. Knopf.

Tilburt, J. C., Emanuel, E. J., Kaptchuk, T. J., Curlin, F. A., & Miller, F. G. (2008, October 23). Prescribing "placebo treatments": results of national survey of US internists and rheumatologists. *The BMJ.* doi:http://doi.org/10.1136/bmj.a1938

Tipler, F. J. (1994). *The Physics of Immortality: Modern Cosmology, God and the Resurrection of the Dead.* New York, USA: Doubleday Publishers.

Urry, J. (2003). *Global Complexity*. Cambridge, Massachuesetts, USA: Polity.

Verhoeven, J. E., Révész, D., Picard, M., Epel, E. E., Wolkowitz, O. M., Matthews, K. A., Puterman, E. (2017, March 28). Depression, telomeres and mitochondrial DNA: between- and within-person associations from a 10-year longitudinal study. *Molecular Psychiatry*. doi:10.1038/mp.2017.48

von Glasenapp, H. (1991). *Die Fünf Weltreligionen*. München: Eugen Diederichs Verlag.

Walsch, N. D. (1997). *Conversations with God* (Vol. 1). London: Hodder and Stoughton.

Walsch, N. D. (1998). *Conversations with God* (Vol. 2). London: Hodder and Stoughton.

Walsch, N. D. (1999). *Conversations with God* (Vol. 3). London: Hodder & Stoughton.

Watts, D. (2003). *Six Degrees: The Science of a Connected Age*. London: Heinemann.

Wellman, B. (Ed.). (1999). *Networks in the Global Village*. Wrestview Press.

Wenger, E. (1998). *Communities of Practice*. Cambridge University Press.

Wheatley, M., & Kellner-Rogers, M. (1998, April). Bringing Life to Organizational Change. *Journal of Strategic Performance Measurement*.

Wheeler, J. A. (1990). Information, Physics, Quantum: The Search for Links. In W. Zurek (Ed.), *Complexity, Entropy, and the Physics of Information*. Redwood City, California, USA: Addison-Wesley.

Whitehead, A. N. (1960, reprint). *Process and Reality*. London: Harper & Row.

Wilber, K. (2001). *A Theory of Everything*. London: Shambhala Publications.

Wilks, Y. (Ed.). (2010). *Close engagements with artificial companions : key social, psychological, ethical and design.* Philadelphia, USA: John Benjamins Publishing.

Winograd, T. (1975). Frame Representations and the Declarative Procedural Controversy. In D. Bobrow, & A. Collins (Eds.), *Representation and Understanding.* New York: Academic Press.

Woodhouse, M. B. (1996). *Paradigm Wars: Worldviews for a New Age.* Berkeley: Frog Books.

Yehuda, R., Daskalakis, N. P., Bierer, L. M., Bader, H. N., Klengel, T., Holsboer, F., & Binder, E. B. (2016, September 1). Holocaust Exposure Induced Intergenerational Effects on FKBP5 Methylation. *Biological Psychiatry, 80*(5), pp. 372-380. Retrieved from http://www.biologicalpsychiatryjournal.com/article/S0006-3223(15)00652-6/fulltext

Zeleny, M. (2006). Knowledge-information Autopoietic Cycles: Towards the Wisdom Systems. *International Journal of Management and Decision Making, 7*(1), 3-18.